Lassine Bagayogo

Epidemiological and therapeutic aspects of diabetes in the elderly

Lassine Bagayogo

Epidemiological and therapeutic aspects of diabetes in the elderly

ScienciaScripts

This book is a translation from the original published under ISBN 978-620-6-70170-5.

Publisher:
Sciencia Scripts
is a trademark of
Dodo Books Indian Ocean Ltd. and OmniScriptum S.R.L publishing group

120 High Road, East Finchley, London, N2 9ED, United Kingdom
Str. Armeneasca 28/1, office 1, Chisinau MD-2012, Republic of Moldova, Europe
Printed at: see last page
ISBN: 978-620-7-79007-4

Contents

DEDICATIONS AND THANKS 2

TRIBUTES TO THE MEMBERS OF THE JURY 5

INTRODUCTION 10

OBJECTIVES 11

PART I 12

PART II 33

PART III 41

PART IV 44

PART V 57

PART VI 60

REFERENCES 61

Appendices 67

DEDICATIONS AND THANKS

Praise be to ALLAH, the All-Merciful, the Most-Merciful, the Omniscient, the Omnipotent, the First and the Last, by whose grace we have been able to carry out this work.

Peace and greetings on the prophet MOHAMMAD and all his family and all the prophets.

I dedicate this work :

To my parents: *Raffa BAGAYOGO and Fatoumata COULIBALY*

Dear parents, this work is yours, this is a way for me to tell you that you can be proud of yourselves, I will never stop thanking you and thanking heaven for having given me parents. The education I received was more than enough to shape the man I have become. I hope to be able to imitate you in the education of my children. May ALLAH give you long life and good health with us and a happy ending.

To my father: *Drissa KEITA*

You have always been there when and where it was needed for me, my brothers and sisters. Humility is your name, dignity and integrity are values that you have always embodied and that you have never ceased to teach us. May ALLAH reward you with goodness and give you long life and health. We pray to GOD to make you proud of us. Once again, thank you!

To my grandmothers: *Iya DIALLO, Assitan COULIBALY and especially to you Aiche MAIGA, you have been a second mother to me, a friend and a confidante. Since I was very young, you have been a source of motivation for me, and you have always taught me to respect family values. May ALLAH help you to make the pilgrimage you so desire and keep you among us in good health.*

To the entire COULIBALY family and the entire BAGAYOGO family:

To all my aunts: *Assitan COULIBALY, Mariam COULIBALY, Aichatou MAIGA, Adja MAIGA, Makoura DOUMBIA, Nassira DIAKITE and Djeneba TRAORE*

To all my maternal uncles: *Yacouba, Drissa and Diakaridia*

To my uncle: *the late Mamadou COULIBALY*

Dear uncle, GOD is not the only witness to everything you have done for me. I would have loved so much for you to see the fruit you have sown, but alas GOD decided otherwise. You have helped me so much during this course of my life, expenses here and there, means of transport, telephones, advice and so on... I cannot mention them all. May ALLAHOURAHMANIRAHEEMI grant you his Paradise, and may he bless your descendants.

To all my paternal uncles: *Sayon, Dioume, LADJI, Dossolo, Sekou, Boubacar and Amadou*

To my brothers: *Chiacka BAGAYOGO, Cheick Oumar BAGAYOGO and Sidy Bekaye COULIBALY*

Thank you so much for your support, may ALLAH strengthen our ties and give us the strength to be able to provide for our family.

To my sirs: *Awa DOUMBIA, Korotouma DOUMBIA, Bintou COULIBALY, Aminata COULIBALY and Tata BAGAYOGO*

To my beloved wives and daughters (Rokia and Assitan): *Sokona TRAORE AND Nastou DIAWARA*

I know that INSHALLAH you will have satisfaction in all that you seek from GOD because of all that you do for the smooth running of this family. I dedicate this work to you and thank you for everything you do, thank you very much!

To my fiancée: *Dr Nafatoumata DIAWARA*

Alhamdoulillah, more than a source of motivation, my alter ego, you have been more than the other half of my head in accomplishing this work. I have not lacked moral and physical support and comfort during this long journey. May ALLAH help us in all our endeavours and give us blessed descendants.

To my wives in ATTbougou: *Babou Bintou Said TOURE and Nana Kadidia DIAWARA*

To my *friends: Malick SIDIBE, Bakary TOGOLA, Djeffla DIALLO, Ousmane TAORE and Mamadou DIALLO*

To my close friends from the 11th numerus clausus class: *Aichata DAO, Yacouba L KONE and Makan OUATTARA*

Dear friends, you have been what we call a second family to me. With you I've never felt lonely and I've never lacked anything. In memory of the good times we've had together and the strong ties that bind us, a big thank you for your encouragement, support and help. With all my affection I wish you every success in everything you do.

To my medical elders: *Dr Sekou LANDOURE, Dr Adama SIDIBE, Dr Moussa DJIRE Dr Mahamadou MALE, Dr Ibrahim MVOUTSI andb Dr Jean Patrick TIENKA.*

Thank you very much dear masters for the quality of the training, I was fully satisfied. May ALLAH reward you with good.

To the PhD students of the Internal Medicine Department of the CHME "Le Luxembourg": *Hamoune SIBY, El Moctar MAIGA. Samba DIARRA, Hamidou KASSAMBARA, Yacouba TAMBOURA, Kadidia MAIGA, Kevine TCHATCHOU*

I'll never stop thanking you, dear colleagues, for everything you've done for me. Thank you for putting up with me and being my partners in everyday life in hospital. I wish you all a very happy career.

To my team on duty in Internal Medicine at CHME "Le Luxembourg": *Amadou DIALLO, Kassim SAMAKE, Bintou KANTE, Dr Mamadou Kalifa GOITA.*

To my team on duty at CSREF CV: *Dr Kadiatou TRAORE, Dr Fatoumata TIERO, Dr Issiacka TRAORE, Adama YANOGUE*

May this work inspire you to greater courage and self-determination. You are called upon to live in a fast-moving world where you have to confront new and ever-increasing problems, and you are obliged to find original solutions to them. The path of life is long and winding. In short, just remember that "man is the baker of his own life". I hope that this work will be an example of courage for you and an incentive to do better.

A special thank you to Dr Kadiatou TRORE, who was always ready to welcome me from the start of my training. May ALLAH accompany you in everything you do.

To Dr Moussa DJIRE:

Throughout the lines of this work, you will find all my gratitude; lost in the midst of my texts, you have vouched for me to ensure the smooth running of this work. Doctor, I will never stop thanking you for what you have done for me. Thank you for everything and enjoy your professional career.

To Professor Modibo SANGARE :

I remember well that day when, after having lost hope, you had to say those words to me through your own journey; and if I have drawn one conclusion from it, it is that: GOD IS CAPABLE OF MAKING YOU CROSS THE DESERT FOR FORTY (40) YEARS SO THAT YOU CAN SAVE OTHER PEOPLE AT THE OTHER END OF THE EARTH. Day and night INSHALLAH, I will never stop praying for you and your descendants. Long life, health and happiness with a good end very dear.

To all the staff of the Internal Medicine Department of the CHME "Le Luxembourg".

To all those who, from near or far, supported me in the realisation of this work
To the entire 11th class of the numerus clausus.
Thank you all so much.

To our Master and thesis president
Professor KAYA Assetou SOUKHO

☐ Full Professor of Internal Medicine at the FMOS

☐ Head of the internal medicine department at the CHU point G ;

☐ Specialist in digestive endoscopy ;

☐ Certificate in applied epidemiology;

☐ Postgraduate diploma in gastroenterology ;

☐ President of the Malian Society of Internal Medicine

☐ Board member of the African Society of Internal Medicine

Dear Master,

Throughout this work, we have greatly appreciated your scientific and human qualities.

It is a great honour for you to chair this jury.

Your teaching in both social and professional life, your rigour in your work, your strong sense of duty, and the deep friendship with your colleagues and students make you a very admirable person.

With this work, we hope to live up to your expectations.

Dear Master, please accept, in all modesty, the expression of our immense gratitude. May the Almighty protect you!

<h1 style="text-align:center">To our Master and director of these
Professor Djibril SY</h1>

- ☐ Member of the Society of Internal Medicine of Mali (SOMIMA)

- ☐ Lecturer in internal medicine at the FMOS;

- ☐ Diploma in geriatric medicine from the University of Rouen and Paris VI in France;

- ☐ Hospital practitioner at the Centre Hospitalier Universitaire (CHU) du Point G

- ☐ Former intern at the Bamako hospitals

Dear Master

We very much appreciated the spontaneity with which you agreed to supervise this work. This shows not only your interest in this work but also your constant concern for the students. Your simplicity and generosity have left their mark on us throughout this work, as you have never put up any barriers between us... Please accept, dear Master, our sincere thanks.

To our Master and Co-Director of Thesis
Professor MENTA Djenebou TRAORE

- ☐ Associate Professor of Internal Medicine at the FMOS

- ☐ Member of the Society of Internal Medicine of Mali

- ☐ Member of the Algerian Society of Internal Medicine

- ☐ Hospital practitioner at CHU du Point G

- ☐ Diploma from the University of Paris VI on the management of HIV

- ☐ Postgraduate training in hepato-gastro-enterology Mohamed V Morocco
Holder of a university diploma (DU) in sickle cell anaemia FMOS

Dear Master
You have done us the honour of co-directing this work,
Your availability, your humility, your modesty and your charisma have always
been appealing human values for us, right from the first moment we met.
You have taught us not only scientific knowledge, but also the principles of
social life, because you have set up no barriers between us.
We would like to express our deepest gratitude.

To our Master and Member of the Jury
Dr Fofana Youssouf

☐ Specialist in internal medicine ;

☐ Diploma in diabetology; Diploma in sickle cell anaemia ;

☐ General Secretary of the Internal Medicine Society of Mali ;

☐ Member of the Malian Society of Endocrinology, Metabolic Disease, Nutrition and Diabetology;

☐ Board member of the African Society of Internal Medicine (SAMI)
Head of Internal Medicine at the CHME Luxembourg;
Dear Master, Your experience, the breadth of your knowledge, your scientific rigour and your dynamism make you an accomplished, admirable and universally respected teacher. Despite your busy schedule, you have never ceased to follow this work. If this work has been possible, we owe it to your determination and sense of responsibility. Many thanks. May the Almighty grant you long life.

To our Master and jury member Dr Kaly KEITA

☐ Internist

☐ In charge of research

☐ Hospital practitioner in the Internal Medicine Department of the Centre Hospitalier du Point (CHU) du Point G

☐ Former head of general medicine at the Fousseyni Daou regional hospital in kayes

☐ Member of SOMIMA and SAMI

Dear Master

The great honour you have done us by agreeing to sit on this jury gives us the opportunity to express our admiration and deep respect. Your simplicity and your availability have left their mark on us.

Please accept our sincerest thanks.

INTRODUCTION

Diabetes mellitus, more simply called diabetes, is a group of metabolic diseases characterized by hyperglycëmia resulting from defects in the secretion or action of insulin, or both[1] .

According to the WHO, a person is considered old if they are at least 65 years old [2] . In Mali, a person is considered old when they are under 60. Geriatrics is the medicine of the elderly, unlike gerontology, which refers to the study of ageing in all its dimensions, including social, economic, demographic, psychological, anthropological, cultural, medical and others [3]. In geriatrics, a geriatric patient is defined as someone aged over 75, most often with multiple pathologies, at high risk of losing their autonomy or becoming increasingly dependent [3].

Worldwide, the vast majority - at least 90% - of diabetic states are caused by a long-standing asymptomatic disease, which typically occurs after the age of 50, particularly in overweight people or those with a family history of the same disease: this is type 2 diabetes (T2D). In the elderly, there is a much rarer, slow-onset type 1 (LADA) and, more generally, what is known as secondary diabetes. Data from a diabetes prevalence study carried out in 146 countries, covering 90% of the world's adult population, shows that between 1980 and 2014, the age-adjusted prevalence of diabetes rose from 4.3% to 9.0% in men and from 5.0% to 7.9% in women, an increase from 108 million in 1980 to 422 million in 2014 [4].

According to the IDF, the prevalence of diabetes increases with age, with the highest estimated prevalence in the over-65s. In 2019, the estimated number of people living with diabetes aged 65 to 99 was 135.6 million (19.3%). If this trend continues, the number of people aged over 65 (65 to 99) living with diabetes will be 195.2 million in 2030 and 276.2 million in 2045. These data point to a significant increase in the number of people living with diabetes in the ageing population over the coming years, and highlight the inevitable public health and economic challenges that this implies [5].

Africa will see the largest increase in diabetes in the world, rising from 19.4 million in 2019 to 47.1 million in 2045 among people aged 65 to 69. The burden of diabetes has therefore already largely shifted to middle- and low-income countries, which raises serious concerns about the ability of these countries to cope with this "epidemic", both in terms of prevention and management[4].

In Mali, the incidence of the disease is estimated at 2.4%, with a progression curve similar to that of the continent in 2045[6] .

Vu l'ampleur que prend la pathologie le diabete du sujet aдë en terme de prevalence, de dëpenses et de morbimortalitU dans le monde ainsi que dans notre pays, avec le caractere de probleme majeur de santë publique dans le monde durant le 3eme millUnaire que lui a attribuéU l'OMS et le fait qu'il n^hait beaucoup d^tude sur le diabete chez le sujet aдë, we considered it necessary to carry out this study with the aim of determining the hospital frequency of diabetic patients as well as the clinical and therapeutic particularities of diabetes in these patients in the internal medicine department of the CME le Luxembourg.

General objective :

To study the epidemiological, clinical and therapeutic aspects of diabëte in *older* subjects in the internal medicine department of the Mëre-Enfant hospital centre (CHME) le Luxembourg in Bamako.

Specific objectives :

> Determining the hospital frequency of diabetes in older people

> Describe the clinical features of diabëte in the elderly;

> Assessing the elderly according to the Global Geriatric Assessment for therapeutic adaptation

> Describing the management of diabetes in the elderly

1. GENERAL

1.1 Definition :

Diabetes is a hëtërogëne group of mëtabolic diseases characterisedërisë by chronic hyperglycëmia resulting from a defect in the secretion and/or action of insulin that can lead to long-term micro and macroangiopathic complications in relation to gënëtic and environmental factors [7].

1.2 Diagnostic criteria :

As diabetes has evolved over time and laboratory diagnostic techniques and resources have advanced, several criteria have been adopted for diagnosing diabetes. Today, based on both blood glucose levels and HbAlc, a subject is considered to have diabetes if he or she is in one of the following situations:

■ Fasting blood glucose greater than or equal to 1.26 g/L (7 mmol/L), defined as no calorie intake for at least 8 hours;

■ Or clinical signs of hyperglycaemia, detected at any time of the day with a blood glucose level of 2 g/L (11.1 mmol/L) or more, regardless of the distance of the blood sample from a meal. The symptoms of hyperglycaemia, when sufficiently marked, are the classic cardinal signs: polyuria, polydipsia, unexplained weight loss often associated with polyphagia;

■ Or blood glucose at the 2nd hour of an OGTT greater than or equal to 2 g/L (11.1 mmol/L). The test should be performed in accordance with WHO (World Health Organisation) recommendations using an oral load of anhydrous glucose equal to 75 g dissolved in water;

■ Or HbAlc greater than or equal to 6.5%.

> In addition, the following are defined:

■ All subjects with a fasting blood glucose between 1 g/L and 1.25 g/L are considered to have an "abnormal fasting blood glucose";

■ Subjects with glucose intolerance are defined as all subjects whose fasting blood glucose level is less than 1.26 g/L and whose blood glucose level at the 2nd hour of an oral hyperglycemia test (75 g of glucose per os) is between 1.40 g/L and 1.99 g/L;

■ All subjects with an HbAlc of between 5.7 and 6.4% [8] are considered to be at "high risk of sugar diabetes".

Glycaemia has both intra- and inter-individual variability. For a fasting glycaemia of 1.26 g/L, it has been shown that the biological variability coefficient of glycaemia, which incorporates both intra- and inter-individual variability, is of the order of 6.9%. HbAlc, on the other hand, has a much lower variabil^. This is why the ADA expert group insisted that it should be included among the diagnostic criteria. Since glycaemia and HbAlc can vary in the same individual, from one day to the next or from one sample to the next, the diagnosis of diabetes mellitus should never be based on a single measurement. Thus, if hyperglycëmia is not obvious from the first visit or from the first test, these criteria must be confirmed by a new test some time later. For example, the discovery of a fasting blood glucose level of 1.40 g/L, i.e. tegereously higher than 1.26 g/L, means that a new fasting blood sample should be taken a few days later to confirm this result[9].

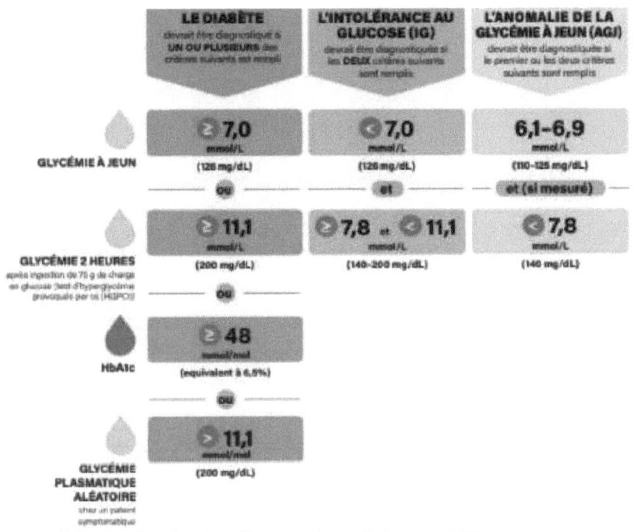

Figure 1: Modified criteria for diagnosing diabetes [5].

1.3 Diabetes classification :

The classification of diabetes has changed very little. **In 1999,** the new WHO recommendations proposed removing the designations "insulin-dependent" and "non-insulin-dependent" and retaining only the terms **"type 1" and "type 2",** dëtaⅢanting the different forms of "other types of diabetes", while continuing to individualise gestational diabetes [10].

1.4 Pathophysiology of diabetes:

1.4.1. Type 1 diabetes

Type 1 diabetes, an autoimmune disease (in 90% of cases and idiopathic in 10%), specific to в-pancreatic cells, is a concept that is barely 40 years old. In the 1970s, the discovery of new markers such as anti-Islet Cell Antibody (ICA) detected by indirect immunofluorescence on human pancreas sections by Bottazzo [11] and major histocompatibility complex (MHC) molecules associated with diabetes by the Nerup group [12] led to the nosographic classification of this form of diabetes and its current name of type 1 diabetes. T1DM accounts for **5-10%** of cases of diabetes [13]. It is most often discovered before the age of 35 and is characterised by the cardinal syndrome of polyuria, polydipsia, weight loss and polyphagia. It may be revealed abruptly by cetoacidosis [14]. Pathophysiologically, it is characterised by absolute insulin deficiency due to destruction of the в cells of the islets of Langerhans by an autoimmune process. In the majority of cases, the role of environmental factors (viruses, changes in intestinal flora, diet) has been suggested. A genetic predisposition is involved. A family history is found in 10% of cases. In 30% of cases, it is associated with other organ-specific autoimmune diseases (Basedow's disease, Hashimoto's thyroiditis, slow adrenal insufficiency due to cortical retraction, Biermer's disease, celiac disease, vitiligo) which are classified as autoimmune polyendocrine syndromes [15].

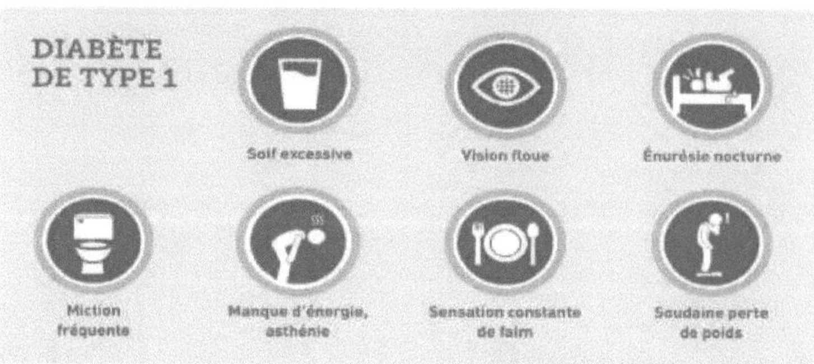

Figure 2: Typical symptoms of type 1 diabetes [5].

1.4.2. Type 2 diabetes :

The 'common' form of type 2 diabetes is a multifactorial disease, an interface between tissue resistance to the action of insulin, a deleterious consequence of so-called modern civilisation, and the inability, genetically transmitted or acquired in the early stages of life, of the в cells of the pancreas to compensate for the increase in the body's insulin requirements that results directly from this. The role of impaired insulin secretion and the interrelationships between insulinopenia and insulin resistance are currently better understood [7].

Insulin resistance :

Insulin resistance is defined as the reduced action of insulin on the target tissues, muscle, liver and adipose tissue. Long-standing studies using the hyperinsulinemic euglycemic clamp method have shown that in patients with type 2 diabetes, glucose uptake by peripheral tissues, particularly muscle, was reduced compared with non-diabetic subjects at identical insulin concentrations [16]. The reduced action of insulin on its target tissues is not responsible for diabetes if it occurs in isolation, without a deficit in insulin production [17], and two situations are physiological: pregnancy (gestational diabetes predicted by insulin resistance in the 2nd trimester of pregnancy) and ageing, which favours type 2 diabetes due to a reduction in muscle mass, which is responsible for an increase in insulin requirements.

Mechanisms of insulin resistance

The mëchanisms by which increased adipose mass decreases the action of insulin at whole-body level are numerous [18]: sëcrëtion of cytokines such as TNF-a, interleukin 6, resistin, Kbëra^on excessive free fatty acids in the circulation by adipose tissue. Muscular insulin resistance is the feature common to all type 2 diabëtics. The mechanisms ëvoquédës to explain it have successively implicated glucose transporters (reduction in their number or affinity), glycogen synthesis and activation of glycogen synthase. This last anomaly, located downstream of the insulin receptor, certainly represents one of the first mechanisms of the disease. Other sites of insulin resistance are the adipocyte and the liver. Circulating lipids are ëlevës in type 2 diabetes and are ëgalement a dëterminating factor in insulinoresistance]. Free fatty acids reduce muscular uptake of glucose and increase its production by the liver. At adipocyte level, insulin's inability to inhibit lipolysis is responsible for an increase in free fatty acids, which stimulate nëoglucogenëse, triglyceride synthesis and glucosëe hëpatic production. The free fatty acids are then used by the muscle, where they reduce glucose uptake and metabolism, and by the pancreas, where they alter insulin secretion (the concept of "lipotoxicity"). In the liver, insulin resistance results in inappropriate glucose output, even in the presence of hyperglycaemia, because hepatic glucose production is less inhibited.

. Genetic determinants of insulin resistance

There are genetic determinants that control energy metabolism, i.e. in practice the greater or lesser susceptibility to developing excess weight in a given nutritional situation. These factors thus modulate insulin sensitivity [19].

. Alteration of insulin secretion :

A deficit in insulin secretion is the common denominator of all forms of diabetes. Impaired insulin secretion, or insulin dysfunction, can take five forms: **pulsatility abnormalities, kinetic abnormalities, qualitative abnormalities, quantitative abnormalities and progressive abnormalities.**

Pulsatility abnormality :

Insulin, like many hormones, is sëcrëtëed in the basal state in a pulsatile mode, with peaks every **10 to 15 minutes** superimposed on a 'background' of wider, slower oscillations, the përiodicitë of which is **60 to 120 minutcs** [20]. The pulsatile mode is the most active in mëtabolic terms. In type 2 diabetes, there is a decrease or disappearance of the rapid oscillatory sëcrëtion of insulin, an anomaly already present in the initial stages of the disease [21-22]. Similarly, a **40%** reduction in the quanta of insulin iK'cessary to maintain normal glycëmia has been observed in patients with type 1 diabëte by switching from continuous to pulsatile administration [23].

Cinetic anomaly :

Although the second phase of 1 insuinosëcrëtion accounts for most of the insulin sëcrëtëe, the early phase is crucial for the control of glycëmia and acts as a signal, 'priming' the liver and allowing increased glucose clearance. The disappearance of the early phase of insulinosëcrëtion after intravenous administration of glucose is a classic doniK'e, dëcrited for more than **30 years** by Cerasi in patients with type 2 diabëte [24]. This anomaly has been confirmed by many authors [25-26]. The precocious phase disappears as soon as fasting glycëmia dëpasses **1.15 g/L** [27].

Qualitative and quantitative anomalies :

The spëcific assay of insulin and its precursors (immunoradiomëtric mëthod or IRMA) described by the Hales group [28] unambiguously demonstrated the patent dëficit of 1 insuinosëcrëtion during type 2 diabëte and settled the controversy of a ëventuel "hyperinsulinism" in type 2 diabëte. Patients with type 2 diabëte have frank insulinopënia at l'ëtat basal and after glucose loading, whether they are of normal weight or obëses [29-30]. On the other hand, there is an abnormal hype^cretion of proinsulin and immature peptides such as, in particular, proinsulin clixre in 32-33 (40% by b cells whereas it accounts for only 5% in the tëmoin non-diëtic subject [31]).

Evolving anomaly :

Insulinosëcrëtion in patients with type 2 diabetes is characterizedërisëe by a progressive reduction over time and by its programmed drying up. Longitudinal studies [32,33] have demonstrated a gradual reduction in insulin secretion, while insulin sensitivity remained at its initial reduced level but did not worsen . From being non-insulin-dependent, type 2 diabetes then became insulin-requiring or insulin-requiring over time, i.e. insulin became necessary to control hyperglycemia. The explanation that seems most relevant to explain the progressive death of в cells is the toxic role of free radicals, produced in excës in the event of hyperglycemia, and the apoptosis of в cells [34,35].

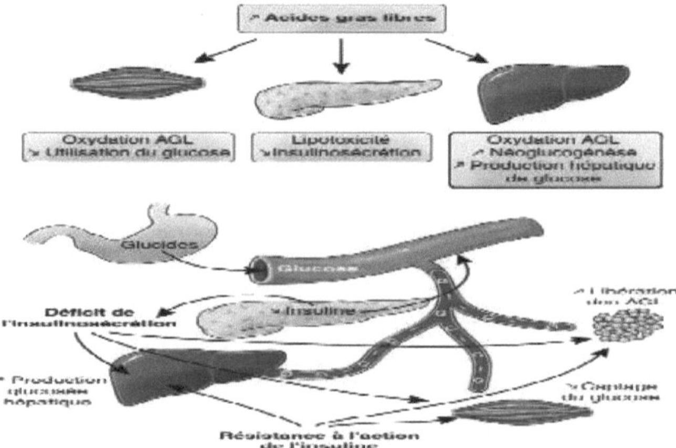

Figure 3: Impact of abnormal insulin secretion and insuiinosensibiiitë in type 2 diabetes [7].

1.4.3. Gestational diabetes :

According to the WHO and the Fëdëration internationale de gynecologie et d'obstëtrique (FIGO), hyperglycëmia during pregnancy can be classified as gestational diabetes (GD) or diabetes in pregnancy (DIP) [36,37]. Gestational diabetes is first diagnosed during pregnancy and can occur at any time during pregnancy (most likely after 24 weeks) [38]. OGTT is recommended for screening for gestational diabetes between 24 and 28 weeks of pregnancy, but for women at high risk, screening should be performed earlier in pregnancy [39].

The criteria for high risk can be listed as follows:

- Obësitë sëvëre ;
- antëcëdents of gestational diabëte or тёre having had an overweight child at birth;
- Presence of glycosuria ;
- Diagnosis of polycystic ovary syndrome;
- Family history of sugar diabetes. The 'increased' risk of gestational diabetes is therefore reduced by the presence of one of the above-mentioned factors.

1.5 Complications of diabetes :

They are classified as acute and chronic complications

1.5.1. Acute complications :

Classically, there are four (4) of these, the first two of which are due to the involution of diabëte, while the last two are iatrogenic.

Diabetic cetoacidosis :

Diabetic c'toacidosis is a life-threatening metabolic complication with a mortality rate of around 5%. It can occur in both type 1 and type 2 diabetics. In T1DM, it may be the cause of disease reversal in 15 to 67% of cases. Insulin deficiency leads to an increase in hepatic gluconeogenesis, glycogenolysis and the release of counter-regulatory hormones (glucagon, cat'cholamines, cortisol, growth hormone). The result is a production of glucose which is not used by the target tissues (muscle, liver, adipose tissue), leading to hyperglycemia. This hyperglycemia leads to osmotic polyuria, which is responsible for dehydration. Functional renal failure sets in, limiting glucose elimination. Insulin deficiency and elevated counter-regulatory hormones also promote lipolysis of triglycerides into free fatty acids. These fatty acids are transformed into tonic bodies in the liver. C'togenesis results in the synthesis of в-hydroxybutyric acid and acetoacetic acid. These acids are eliminated via the urinary and respiratory tracts. Their accumulation leads to the development of metabolic acidosis, which is aggravated by renal failure. Clinically, a distinction is made between 2 phases; the c'tose phase associating the cardinal signs of major diabetes and a digestive picture (nausea, vomiting, abdominal pain) and a c'toacidosis phase comprising Kussmaul's dyspnoea, predominantly extracellular dehydration and consciousness disorders. Actual coma occurs in less than 10% of cases. Biological tests reveal hyperglycëmia (> 2.50 g/l), cëtonëmia > 5 mmol/1 and cëtonuria ++ at ++++. Treatment is based on rehydration, insulin therapy, correction of liydro-electrolvatic disorders and treatment of a ëventuel dëclenchant factor [40].

. Hyperosmolar coma :

Type 2 diabetes is less common than cetoacidosis, but has a higher mortality rate of around 20%. This mortality rate is attributable to the fragility of the patient's condition, complications and poor management. In physiopathological terms, hyperosmolarity results from the combination of insulinopenia and ëlëvation of counter-regulatory hormones. This leads to stimulation of neoglucogenesis, glycogënolyse and a decrease in përiphëric glucose consumption leading to hyperglycemia. Hyperglycaemia in turn leads to osmotic diuresis resulting in dehydration. Functional renal failure sets in, aggravating the hyperglycaemia and establishing hypernatremia. The cells, lacking glucose, turn to lipid metabolism. However, enough insulin is produced to block lipolysis and cetogenesis [41]. Hyperosmolarity develops over several days in a particular type of patient (age >70 years, unrecognised diabetes, diabetes not treated with insulin, cognitive disorders, treatment with certain drugs such as corticosteroids, diurctics, в blockers) in the presence of a triggering factor in 80% of cases (infections, myocardial infarction, stroke, medical or surgical illness). Symptoms include dehydration, which progressively leads to asthenia and weight loss, and consciousness disorders leading to coma, sometimes accompanied by convulsions. Cardiovascular collapse may also occur. Biological tests show blood glucose >6g/l, rising to 15g/l, plasma osmolarity >350 mosm/l, corrected natremia >150 mmol/l, and hypercrcatincmia [42] Management is based on rehydration, insulin therapy, correction of electrolyte disorders, antibiotic therapy if necessary after taking blood samples, and prevention of thromboembolic diseases [43].

Hypoglycemic coma :

Hypoglycaemia is defined as a blood glucose level <3.9mmol/L (0.7 g/L). It affects both type 1 and type 2 diabetics treated with insulin, sulphonylurea or, more rarely, biguanide [44]. In healthy subjects, a fall in glycaemia leads to a fall in insulinemia and an increase in counter-regulatory hormones. The fall in insulinemia results in an increase in glucose synthesis by the liver and a reduction in its use by the target tissues (muscle and adipose tissue). The increase in glucagon stimulates glvcogënolvse. Adrenalin also stimulates glucose synthesis. In diabetics, these defence mechanisms may be altered, leading to hypoglycaemia [45]. Hypoglycaemia, at around 3.6-3.9 mmol/L, is manifested by neurovegetative signs (sweating, palpitations, tremors, hunger) and neuroglycopenic signs (concentration or mood disorders, speech difficulties, incoordination, diplopia, behavioural disorders) when blood glucose levels are around 3mmol/L. It can progress to coma with convulsions [46]. In practice, the ADA has proposed classifying hypoglycemia into severe hypoglycemia, documented symptomatic hypoglycemia, asymptomatic hypoglycemia and relative hypoglycemia [45]. Minor hypoglycemia is managed by eating 3 lumps of sugar or 3 spoonfuls of jam, whereas hypoglycemia with impaired consciousness requires intravenous injections of glucose or intramuscular injections of glucagon [47].

Lactic acidosis :

Lactic acidosis is an organic metabolic acidosis due to an accumulation of lactic acid by an increase in its production or a decrease in its utilisation [48]. Lactic acid results from the conversion of pyruvate during glycolysis. In aerobic conditions, there is a balance between tissue release of lactic acid and its uptake by the liver and kidney. In a situation of hypoxia or acute circulatory disturbance or elimination failure (renal and hepatic failure) in type 2 diabetics using metformin, this balance is lost in favour of lactic acid, resulting in hyperlactatemia. This hyperlactatemia may exceed the hepatic and renal uptake capacities, leading to the development of metabolic acidosis. The clinical picture begins with asthenia, muscle cramps and abdominal or chest pain. Once the acidosis has set in, there are disturbances of consciousness, polypnoea, tachycardia, a fall in blood pressure and oliguria. If left untreated, the patient progresses to shock. Biological tests show

These include metabolic acidosis pH<7.3; high anion gap-12 mmol/l; lactateëmia> 7mmol /l; glycaemia may be elevated, normal or decreased; and functional liyperkalemic renal failure [49]. It is based on extrarenal purification. Prevention requires compliance with the contraindications and precautions for use of metformin [48].

1.5.2. Chronic complications of diabetes:

The chronic complications of diabëte are:

- Damage to the blood vessels,

- Muscles,

and nerves, occurring during long-term revolution of diabëte. There are two types, microangiopathies (damage to the eyes, kidneys and nerves) and macoangiopathies (damage to the heart, arteries of the brain and lower limbs).

Microangiopathic complications :

Ocular diseases: Diabetes-related ocular diseases are a particularly dreaded complication of diabetes, and essentially include diabetic retinopathy (DR), diabetic macular retinopathy (DMR), cataract and glaucoma, but also diplopia and inability to focus.

- Diabetic retinopathy: DR

It is the leading cause of blindness in people aged 20 to 60 in developed countries: 2% of diabetics go blind and 10% become partially sighted [50]. In 2019, a systematic review[51] of the incidence of DR based on eight studies carried out after 2000 (five in Asia, one in North America, one in the Caribbean and one in sub-Saharan Africa) found that the annual incidence of DR ranged from 2.2% to 12.7% and that the annual progression to vision-threatening DR was 3.4% to 12.3%.The risk and aggravating factors for diabetic retinopathy are the length of time diabetes has been progressing, poor diabetic control and too rapid glycemic control, hypertension, cataract surgery, dyslipidëmia, puberty and pregnancy[52]. While certain visual problems may indicate the presence of diabetic retinopathy (dëformëed letters when reading, difficulty switching from light to dark...), retinopathy remains silent for

many years and clinical signs only appear at the stage of complications (néo retinal vascularisation, macular redëme). Any drop in visual acuity corresponds to very advanced lesions that evolve at a low level. It therefore associates two types of lesions:
- Retinal capillary occlusions, the cause of retinal ischaemia, and its complication, pre-retinal neovascularisation.
- The rupture of the internal hemato-retinal barrier, a source of diffusion, leading to macular scarring. While treatments exist and are effective in slowing the progress of the disease and preventing blindness, the best treatment remains prevention through regular check-ups (at least once a year) with an ophthalmologist. Glycemic balance, controlled blood pressure and a healthy lifestyle also help to slow the progression of the disease.
Classification of diabetic retinopathy :
- **Stage 1:** non-proliferative **RD** (<u>minimal</u>: micro-aneurysms; <u>moderate</u>: punctiform haemorrhages, dysuric nodules; <u>severe</u>: (pre-proliferative) : AMIR, patchy hemorrhage
- **Stage 2:** Uncomplicated proliferative **DR** >preretinal and pre-papillary neovaisseau, or complicated > intravitreal haemorrhage, retinal detachment by traction, neovascular glaucoma which may progress on its own despite treatment.

> **Maculopathy:** Can be seen at all stages.
>iscliemique
>Focal redundant
>diffuse redistribution

> **Glaucoma:** Neovascular due to intraocular hypertonia

> **Cataracts:** precocious, 4 to 10% of young diabetics

. Diabetic nephropathy :
Diabetic nephropathy is defined by the persistent presence of albuminuria in the presence of diabetes, more or less associated with an alteration in creatinine clearance [53]. Diabetes is the leading cause of chronic end-stage renal disease. Its prevalence is 60% in the United States and almost 40% in Europe [54]. Worldwide, more than 80% of end-stage renal disease is due to diabetes, hypertension or a combination of the two. The percentage of end-stage renal disease attributed to diabetes ranges from 10% to 67% [55]. Moreover, the prevalence of end-stage renal disease is up to 10 times higher in people living with diabetes than in the rest of the population. Approximately 50% of people with diabetes will develop nephropathy during their lifetime [56]. The main risk factors for diabetic nephropathy are a long history of diabetes and chronic poor glycemic and blood pressure control. Other factors have been suggested: smoking, dyslipidemia, proteinuria, glomerular hyperfiltration and diet [57].renal damage in elderly diabetics is rarely purely glomerular but more often multifactorial. If renal function deteriorates, obstructive uropathy should always be considered, particularly in men, in whom a rectal examination should be performed as a matter of course. Screening for diabetic nephropathy is recommended five years after the discovery of T1DM. For T2DM, screening should be carried out as soon as diabetes is diagnosed, as 7% of this group of patients already have microalbuminuria at the time of diagnosis [57]. The diagnosis of diabetic nephropathy is based on the discovery of albuminuria confirmed on two occasions by three urine tests taken one to eight weeks apart.
Pathological microalbuminuria is a predictive factor for cardiovascular mortality and morbidity

Classification of diabetic nephropathyj
Diabetic nephropathy evolves in 5 stages **(Mogensen classification)** [58].
* **Stage 1:** Functional nephropathy **(from the onset of diabetes)**
Normal EUA (<30mg/24h), normal BP
* **Stage 2:** Silent (latent) kidney disease **(after 2 to 6 years)**
Normal or elevated stress EUA, normal BP
* **Stage 3:** Beginning nephropathy (incipient) **(7 to 15 years)**
Presence of permanent micro proteinuria: EUA 30-300mg/24h; normal or high BP.
* **Stage 4:** Acquired kidney disease **(after 15 years)**
EUA>300mg/24h >macro   proteinuria>nephrotic syndrome,
Hypertension and retinopathy
* **Stage 5:** End-stage renal failure **(7 to 15 years)**
Constant hypertension, ^Glomerular filtration
Dialysis required
Diabetic neuropathy :
Diabetes is the leading cause of neuropathy worldwide. Its prevalence varies from 8 to 60% depending on the study, and increases with the duration of diabetes. In addition, 7.5% of patients develop symptomatic neuropathy as soon as their diabetes is diagnosed. It affects both the autonomic and peripheral nervous systems [59]. The main risk factors are the duration of the disease and poor diabetic control, as in nephropathy and diabetic retinopathy. Other factors such as age over 50, male sex, tall stature, alcoholism, chronic hypoxia, nutritional factors, arterial ischaemia of the lower limbs and too rapid glycaemic control have been suggested [60]. Chronic hyperglycaemia leads to the conversion of glucose into sorbitol, which accumulates in the cell. This accumulation of sorbitol leads to a decrease in the activity of the sodium-potassium adenosine triphosphatase pump (Na+/K+ATPase), resulting in a slowdown in conduction velocity. Glycation also leads to the formation of advanced glycation products (AGEs), which denature proteins in the nervous system. The increase in free radicals is at the root of oxidative stress. The Brown and Asbury classification allows neuropathies to be divided into four types:
Distal and symmetrical neuropathies
Symmetrical proximal motor neuropathies
Focal and multifocal neuropathies
Autonomic neuropathy (digestive tract neuropathy, vësical neuropathy, genital neuropathy, cardiac autonomic neuropathy,...)
The aim of treatment is to relieve the symptoms of neuropathy. It is based on glycemic control and tricyclic antidepressants, antiepileptics and opiate derivatives. Level 1 analgesics are not very effective [59].
Macoangiopathic complications :
Heart disease :

> **Heart failure :**
Earlier and more sëvëre, often painless:
Silent myocardial ischemia (SMI): 30%.
Painless myocardial infarction (MI): 50 to 70%.
In T1DM, the incidence of cardio ischemic accidents is 5% after the age of 30, and the renal impairment is a major factor In T2DM, the risk is 2 to 3 times higher.

The pathophysiology is a combination of multi-truncular and distal atherosclerotic lesions, moderate stenosis and abnormalities of the coronary microcirculation. The cardiovascular risk is linked to insulin resistance. This syndrome is accompanied by arterial hypertension and lipid disorders: - Decrease in HDL-cholesterol (High Density Lipoproteins-cholesterol), which transports cholesterol to the liver for elimination - Increase in LDL-cholesterol (Low Density Lipoproteins-cholesterol). There are also inflammatory phenomena, probably due to the secretion by fatty tissue of these inflammatory messengers. All these factors are risk factors for developing cardiovascular complications. Sedentary lifestyle, stress and especially smoking can also contribute to these phenomena [33]. Cardiovascular complications are the main cause of death in patients with type 2 diabetes. Cardiovascular morbidity and mortality are multiplied by a factor of 2 to 3 in men and 4 to 5 in women.

> **Cardiac neuropathy :**

It results in resting tachycardia, orthostatic hypotension leading to malaise and syncope or orthostatic stroke, sudden cardiorespiratory arrest during дёпёгаle anaesthesia.

Arteriopathy of the lower limbs:

This is a classic complication of diabёte, usually consideredёrёe as one of the localisations of macroangiopathy. In addition to dёsёquilibre glycёmique, smoking is a powerful risk factor for this condition. There is nothing specific about the clinical signs, but they are rarely isolated and are most often associated with diabёtic neuropathy and infection, which together form the diabёtic foot. It is precocious, rapidly progressive, diffuse, mainly in the leg, and associated with mediacalcosis (calcification of the media).It is either asymptomatic (well compensated), in which case it is a marker of global arterial damage, in which case the proof is represented by the global cardiovascular risk; or symptomatic (Leriche and Fontaine classification), in which case the immediate risk is evaluated by the risk of trophic disorder and amputation.

Leriche and Fontaine classification:
* **stage 1:** Clinical latency
* **stage 2:** Intermittent claudication
* **stage 3:** Decubitus pain
* **stage 4:** Dry or damp gangrene

Cerebral arteriopathy: cerebrovascular accident (CVA)

Due to atherosclerosis of the vessels in the neck (carotid arteries, vertebral arteries), this type of stroke is more ischemic thanmorrhagic. Clinical signs vary, with sudden onset of sensory, motor or sensory-motor deficit.

Arterial Hypertension (AH) :
* Frequent in T2DM:43%.
* Frequent in T1DM with ^phropathy
* Increases the risk of micro and macro angiopathy
* **Each $PAS is associated with a 15% increase in coronary risk.**

Mixed complications :

> **Diabetic foot:**

The concept of the "diabetic foot" covers all the conditions (wounds, deformities, ulcerations) affecting the foot in diabetic patients, directly related to the consёquences of hyperglycёmia. Infection, ulceration or destruction of the deep tissues of the foot associated with neuropathy and/or peripheral arteriopathy of the lower limbs in diabetic patients. Its prevalence ranges from 1.8% to 7.4% [61]. Amputations are 10 to 20 times more frequent in diabetic patients [62].

Every 20 seconds there is an amputation worldwide due to diabetes (1.3 million people with diabetes lose a leg every year).

A classification system can be used to identify patients at risk from foot problems:

S **Grade 0**: absence of sensory neuropathy and arteriopathy

S **Grade 1**: presence of isolated sensitive neuropathy

S **Grade 2**: association of neuropathy with arteriopathy or foot deformities

S **Grade 3**: history of ulceration lasting more than 3 months or amputation.

Neuropathy manifests itself as hypoesthesia and favours osteoarticular deformations. With these deformations, the pressure points are permanently under pressure. The body reacts with hyperkeratosis, which develops into a callus. This callus dissects the soft tissue, forming a sterile collection. The callus can also rupture and form a gateway. The occurrence of a wound on an arteriopathy leads to an increase in the need for local blood flow, which is already at a maximum. This leads to imbalance and necrosis. The necrosis helps to maintain the infection which, when it spreads, extends the necrosis [63].

For clinical practice,

Management is based on glycemic control, removal of pressure, local treatment of the wound, antibiotic therapy if necessary, and updating of anti-tetanus vaccination [63].

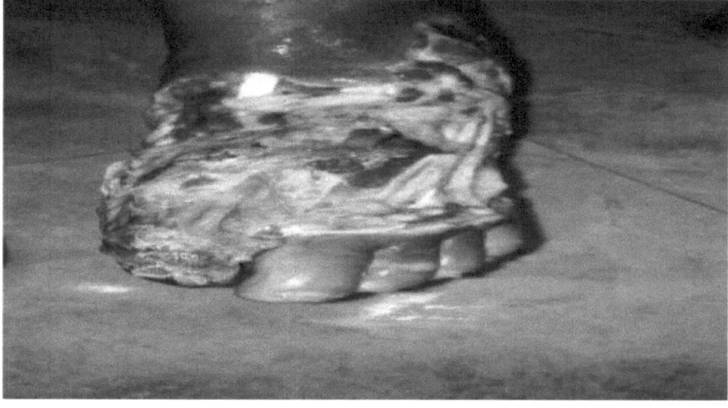

Figure 4: Foot of a diabetic, class D3 according to the Texas classification. **>**

Erectile dysfunction :

Erectile dysfunction (ED) is defined as the persistent or recurrent inability to obtain or maintain an erection permitting satisfactory sexual intercourse [64]. Its prevalence varies with age; its frequency is 32% in T1DM patients and 46% in T2DM patients. Risk factors for ED include diabetes, cardiovascular disease, dyslipidemia, smoking, hormone deficiency and psychological disorders [65]. Management is based on a healthy diet, glycaemic control, treatment of risk factors and specific treatment. This specific treatment is based on phosphodiesterase type 5 inhibitors (Sildenafil, Tadalafil, Vardenafil), local treatments (intracavernosal injections, intraurethral prostaglandin gels) and penile implants [64].

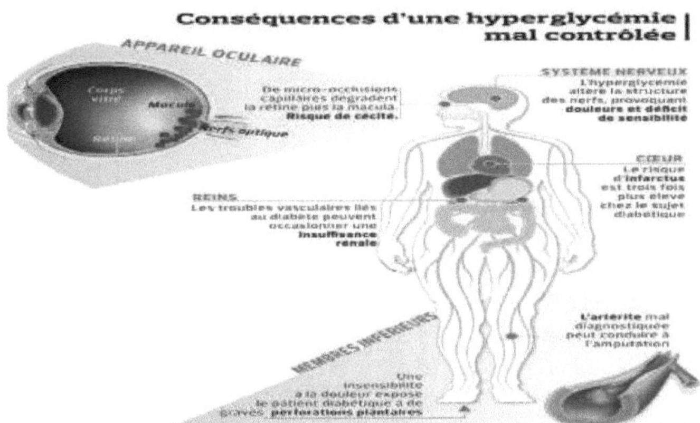

Figure 5: Chronic complications of diabetes [66].

1.6 TREATMENT

1.6.1. Purpose of treatment :

-AшёHorer the diabetic patient's quality of life

-Preventing or treating complications of diabetes

1.6.2. Treatment objectives :

* **General aims of the treatment**
* Reduce the symptoms associated with hyperglycemia and prevent hypoglycemia,
* Detecting, treating and reducing the worsening of diabetes complications,
* Managing associated pathologies to reduce functional disability and improve quality of life,
* Fostering a positive attitude in patients and those around them.

> **Glycemic targets :**

They must be individualised, taking into account :

* Life expectancy (a function of physiological age and associated pathologies),
* The existence of diabetes complications.

Schematically, several situations can be encountered:

* In a patient with long-standing diabetes, there is no need to change the treatment goals in principle. The best possible glycaemic balance should be sought, taking into account the risk of hypoglycaemia (fasting plasma glucose around **1.40 g/l (7.7 mmol/l); with HbA1c around 7.5%).**

* In a person **under 75 years of age without disability,** the discovery of diabetes imposes identical glycemic targets. This approach is justified by the fact that the patient has sufficient life expectancy to develop microangiopathy and that there is a correlation between glycaemic control and cardiovascular mortality.

* In patients aged **over 75** with newly diagnosed diabetes, glycaemic targets should be set on an individual basis, taking into account life expectancy and the risk of hypoglycaemia. Indeed, there are no studies demonstrating the benefits of strict glycaemic control over the age of 75.

* In polypathological patients with a short life expectancy, the aim should be to achieve a

comfort glycemia of **2 g/l (11 mmol/l),** with monitoring to prevent hyperosmolar coma.

1.6.3. Treatment methods :

There are two main types:

Non-pharmacological treatment: Diet and physical activity;

Pharmacological treatment.

Non-pharmacological means

Therapeutic patient education :

According to the WHO, "the purpose of therapeutic education is to train patients to acquire adequate skills to achieve a balance between their lives and optimal control of their disease. Therapeutic patient education is an ongoing process that forms an integral part of medical care. Therapeutic patient education includes awareness, information, learning and psychosocial support, all of which are related to the disease and its treatment. Training should also enable patients and their families to work more effectively with their carers". [67]

> **Hygienic and dietetic regime :**

Although pharmacological treatment is essential in the management of the majority of diabetic patients, most recommendations recognise that hyggiëno-diëtëtic measures remain one of the foundations of diabetes therapy, whether type 1 or type 2. The initial treatment of type 2 diabetes consists of modifying lifestyle habits: diet and physical activity; 80% of type 2 diabetics are obëses. The fight against sëdentaritë, along with a ëq'ulibrëe diet, are therefore the essential foundations of the management of type 2 diabëte.

Given the frequency of weight overload in type 2 diabetes and the pathophysiological role played by the insulin resistance induced by weight overload in type 2 diabetes, we can state that controlling and restricting calorie intake is, in the majority of cases, the common denominator of dietetic measures. Based on this observation, numerous dietetic strategies have been put forward: traditional diets, selectively restrictive diets in carbohydrates or lipids. Weight-loss (low-calorie) diets are based on achieving a balance between calorie intake and energy expenditure, but they often fail because patients find it difficult to cope with the constraints of calorie restriction over the long term. Eating habits should be assessed at the outset using a dietary survey. [68]

• The food survey :

It allows you to specify the calorie level, not forgetting the calories from alcohol, the number of meals eaten per day, and the breakdown between the different nutrients.

• Rëduction in calorie intake:

The aim is to achieve a weight loss of 1 to 4 kg per month. Calorie intake is usually reduced by 20 to 30% compared with the dietary survey data. However, a markedly low-calorie diet is incompatible with a normal social, professional and family life. Under these conditions, it is rare for diabetics to be prescribed a diet of less than 1600 calories for women and 1800 calories for men. Naturally, the calorie level will be adapted to the rate of weight loss and tolerance.

- Breakdown of food intake :

Calorie intake should be spread over at least 3 meals a day. Eating breakfast is important, but often absent in obese people. It is often useful to divide the diet into five portions (3 main meals and 2 snacks) to spread the calorie intake more evenly over the day. Meals and snacks should be mixed. Combining carbohydrates with proteins and lipids makes meals less hyperglycemic.

- Distribution between the different nutrients :

It should be close to the normal distribution:

50-55% carbohydrates,

30-35% fat and

15% protein.

The safety carbohydrate ration to be maintained is at least 100g of carbohydrate per day. The minimum protein intake is 0.7g/Kg/day.

- Carbohydrates: [69] [70]

- Carbohydrates are not essential macronutrients. They should be incorporated into the diet in a sensible and reasonable way. Limiting them is a simple, effective and safe solution to weight control. They are the first source of energy to be reduced when trying to lose weight.

- Avoid or limit carbohydrates with a high glycemic index. They encourage fat storage, stimulate the appetite and increase the risk of diabetes, cardiovascular disease and high blood pressure. They include table sugar, confectionery, Viennese pastries and other baked goods, as well as refined foods such as white bread and breakfast cereals like cornflakes. Fast-absorbing sugars should be avoided, partly because they are hyperglycemic, but also because they provide a significant amount of calories in a small volume. Fruit may be eaten, but only on a limited scale.

Fruit accounts for 5% of the carbohydrate intake, milk for 5% and slow sugars for 90%.

You should try to keep fruit in your diet, bearing in mind that solid foods have a lower glycaemic index than liquid foods (it's better to eat a whole orange than to drink a squeezed orange), and you should encourage the consumption of apples, kiwis and green pears rather than sweeter fruits (bananas, melon, etc.).

- Give priority to carbohydrates with a low or moderate glycemic index. They have the advantage of not causing insulin spikes. Vegetables, which should be eaten in moderation, should form the main part of the carbohydrate intake, as should fruit, one per meal. Other interesting sources of carbohydrates include basmati or wild rice, quinoa, buckwheat, sweet potatoes and other tubers. Pulses can also be an interesting source (always after soaking and/or fermentation, and with gentle cooking). Finally, cereals are not a source to be favoured, in particular 'modern' wheat in all its forms (bread, pasta, etc.) which should be avoided wherever possible. It would be better to prefer its ancestors (small spelt or kamut), or cereals such as millet, barley or oats (preferably semi-complete versions).

- Prefer al dente cooking: To avoid raising the glycemic index of carbohydrates. To sum up, try to eat carbohydrates at every meal, but in reasonable quantities: prefer so-called "slow" sugars such as wholemeal bread, al dente pasta and semi-cereal rice.

- Lipids: [69,70]

Fats are essential to life. We mustn't neglect them, but give priority to good quality fats:

- As far as possible, avoid Trans fatty acids and partially hydrogenated industrial oils (fast food, prepared industrial meals in particular);

- By limiting certain saturated fatty acids (fatty charcuterie such as rillettes, sausages, rosette);

- The consumption of polyunsaturated and monounsaturated fatty acids is favoured over that of saturated fatty acids. You should try to limit excess lipids (one tablespoon of oil per day), and prefer végétal oils to animal fats in order to atёHoгer the отёда 6 / отёда 3 ratio and thus provide a vasoprotective effect.

- And don't forget the omega-9s found in olive oil, macadamia nuts and avocado;

- By deprioritising essential omega-3 fatty acids (oily fish, walnuts, linseed oil), while taking care to reduce consumption of omega-6 (sunflower, soya, mat's, grape seed or safflower oil).

• Alcoholic beverages: These should be reduced because of their high calorie content and the addiction and dependence they entail. They should not exceed one glass of wine per meal.

• Dietary fibres: [71] Their consumption has a double bÏërë! On the one hand they reduce post prandial hyper glycëmic flSche, and on the other they help to combat constipation induced by a hypocaloric diet. Although our bodies are unable to digest them, fibre is vital for our digestive system. As well as playing an important role in the mechanical action of digestion, they are directly involved in the good healthë of our intestinal flora, which itself plays a e!ë role in maintaining our immune system. It is advisable to eat as many tegumes as possible. Tegumineuses can also ëlre an interesting source of fibre (after soaking/fermentation). Last but not least, think about dried nuts (almonds, walnuts, hazelnuts) and mushrooms, which are very rich in в-glucans, which stimulate the immune system as well as being ferments in the intestine.

It's important to opt for wholegrain cereals and organic wholegrain or semi-wholegrain cereal products (wholegrain bread, wholegrain rice, wholegrain pasta), nuts and seeds. The more refined the cereals (and therefore the less complete they are), the lower the fibre content. Fibre is present in oats (flakes, bran, flour), barley, rye, legumes (red or white beans, green or coral lentils, chickpeas, beans), dried figs and prunes. Fruits rich in pectin, such as apples, pears and oranges, and fresh vegetables (carrots, courgettes, asparagus, etc.) also contain pectin, as do seaweeds in the form of alginates. Salads, crudités, compotes or homemade mueslis can be spiced up with nuts and seeds (flaxseed, for example) crushed or ground.

Other tips include :

- Prefer lean meats: chicken, rabbit, veal, white ham, etc.; - Eat vegetables as much as you like, preferably short-cooked (to preserve their vitamin content) and low in fat (season preferably with spices);

- Eat three dairy products a day;

- bear in mind that no food is forbidden (occasional consumption in small quantities is always possible);

- for people undergoing treatment that can lead to hypoglycaemia, always carry foodstuffs that can help to correct it.

> **Physical activity :**

Physical activity can be defined as any movement resulting from the contraction of skeletal muscles and causing energy expenditure in addition to the basal resting energy expenditure. Activity can take a variety of forms: competitive sport, sports training, leisure activities, DIY, gardening, etc. Whatever the context, all physical activities fit in with other therapeutic approaches to diabetes mellitus, such as diStStic measures and pharmacological treatments, whether insulin-based or not. By facilitating the use of glucose and increasing sensitivity to endogenous insulin, physical activity helps to control glycaemia in type 2 diabetics. It also improves dyslipidemia by increasing HDL and reducing triglycsrides. In practice, it is advisable to do three 45-minute sessions a week of more intensive activity adapted to the patient's profile. It maintains the osteoarticular system and helps maintain satisfactory muscle mass, and contributes to general hygiene. Physical exercise must be regular, tailored to the patient's needs, prescribed after a cardiovascular assessment, and involve a degree of relaxation for the patient.

Pharmacological means :

These include insulin and oral antidiabetics (OADs).

Insulin :

Insulin is the essential treatment for type 1 diabetes [72]. This treatment should be started as soon as diabetes mellitus is discovered [73]. In type 2 diabetes, insulin therapy is not compulsory as long as hygienic and diëtëtic measures and treatment with oral antidiabëtics or GLP-1 receptor agonists enable glycaemic control targets to be achieved. However, rinsulinotherapy becomes essential on a chronic basis when the disease ëvolves towards the failure of non-insulin treatments (oral antidiabetics at maximum tolerated doses or GLP-1 analogues [74-75]). In type 2 diabète, transient insulin treatment may be necessary in certain situations: intercurrent pathological states, treatment with corticoids.

> **Principle of dose adjustment :**

The 4 areas of insulin therapy

- **Adjusting wake-up blood glucose levels to** avoid nocturnal hypoglycaemia
- **Triple dose adjustment**
- based on previous giycëmies
- based on current blood glucose (if greater than > 3 g/i = + 2 u)
- in preparation for physical activity (decrease from 2 to 8 u)

> **Keeping the same injection area** at the same time of day

> **Preventing and treating hypoglycemia**

> **Means of injection:** -insulin pens, graduated disposable syringes, insulin pumps

> **Injection sites:** arm, thigh, buttock, abdomen

> **Dose:** 0.1-0.8 units /Kg of body weight per day

> **Side effects:** hypoglycaemia, lipohypertrophy (weight gain).

> **Insulin therapy interactions**: Insulin therapy may be introduced either temporarily to deal with an acute clinical situation, or definitively (more often than not) after oral treatments have failed.

> **Different types of insulin:** The different types of insulin currently available have different kinetics, so that insulin treatment can be adapted to the profile of the diabetic patient.

Tableau I   Insulin classes

Insuline	Exemples	Délai d'action	Durée d'action	Indication
Analogue Ultrarapide	Humalog ® Novorapid ®	5 minutes	3 heures	Repas Urgences
Rapide	Actrapid ®	30 minutes	6 heures	
Intermédiaire	NPH ® Umuline ® Insuman ®	1 heure	12 heures	Insuline basale
Lente	Lantus ® Levemir ®	2 heures	24 heures	
Mélanges	Novomix n ® Umuline profil n ®	Mélange avec n% de rapide, le reste de NPH		

Oral antidiabetics(OADs) :

There are several therapeutic classes:

> **Insulin sensitisers**

Biguanides

> **Insulin secretors**

Sulfonamides

Glinids

Les Incretines

> Glucoside inhibitors

Tableau II   ADO classes

DCI	Trade names and strengths	Main adverse effects	Contraindications
Biguanides Metformin	Glucophage cp (500mg, 850mg, 1000mg) Stagid 700mg cp	Abdominal pain Digestive disorders Allergies Vitamin B12 malabsorption **Lactic acidosis**	Renal insufficiency: risk of hypoxia
Sulfonamides Glibenclamide Gliclazide Glimepiride	Daonil cp (1.25mg, 1.25mg and 5 mg) Diamicron cp (30mg cp LM, 60mg) Amarel cp (1, 2, 3 and 4mg)	Hypoglycemia Weight gain Skin allergies	Renal failure Liver failure
Glinids repaglinide nateglinide	Novonorm cp (0.5mg, 1mg and2mg) Starlix	hypoglycemia Hepatic cholestasis	Renal insufficiency or severe liver disease
Acarbose **glucosidase inhibitors** Miglitol	Glucor 50mg and 100mg Diastabol 50mg and 100mg)	Abdominal pain Flatulence Cytolytic hepatitis	IBD Renal failure with clearance<25ml/min
DPP-4 inhibitors	Januvia 100mg cp,		

Sitagliptin	xelevia 100mg cp		Allergy to one of the components
Vidagliptin	Galvus 50 mg	Nausees rhinopharyngitis	
Saxagliptin	Onglyza 5mg cp		
GLP1 agonists Exenatide dulaglutide Liraglutide **SGLT2 inhibitors**	Byetta (5gg, 10 gg per dose, 2inj/d) Trulicity 0.75mg, 1.5mg suspension for injection Victoza (solution for injection SC at 6mg/ml, 1inj/d) LP forms 1inj/s Dapagliflozin Canagliflozin Empagliflozin Ertugliflozin	Nausees Vomiting Pancreatitis Urogenital tract infections, hypotension, dehydration	Renal insufficiency

Mechanism of action of oral antidiabetics (OADs) :

> Insulinosensitizers :

Only metformin is marketed in Mali. Metformin works by three mechanisms:
-Inhibition of neoglucogenesis and glycogenolysis
-increased sensitivity to insulin
-by delaying intestinal absorption of glucose.

> Insulin blockers (hypoglycemic sulphonamides and glinides):

They act by stimulating the HbёraHon of 1 insulin by the в cells of the pancreatic islets of Langerhans.

> SGLT2 inhibitors :

They inhibit the physiological reabsorption of glucose by reducing the renal glucose threshold to close to 0.80 g/L, resulting in glycosuria. This glycosuria helps to lower blood glucose levels.

> DPP4 inhibitors:

Inhibition of the activity of DPP-4, the GLP-1-dependent enzyme;
Increase in insulin6cretion as a function of glycёmia;
Reduction in postprandial glycaёmia.

> GLP-1 agonists :

Increased sёcrёtion of insulin Hёc a la glycёmie ;
Rёduction of glucagon sёcrёtion;
Slowing of gastric emptying (variable depending on the module) ;
Increased satiёtё, reduced food intake (variable depending on the individual) modules).

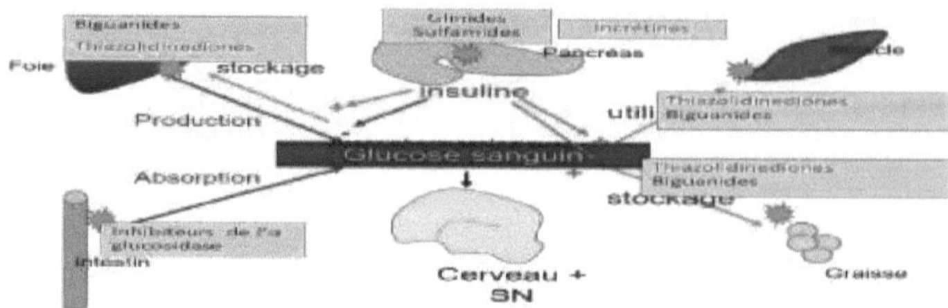

Figure 6: Mechanism of action of antidiabetics [76].

1.6.4. Therapeutic indications :
Type 1 diabetes: lifelong insulin treatment
Type 2 diabetes: medical strategy for glycaemic control of type 2 diabetes
HAS, 2013 [77].

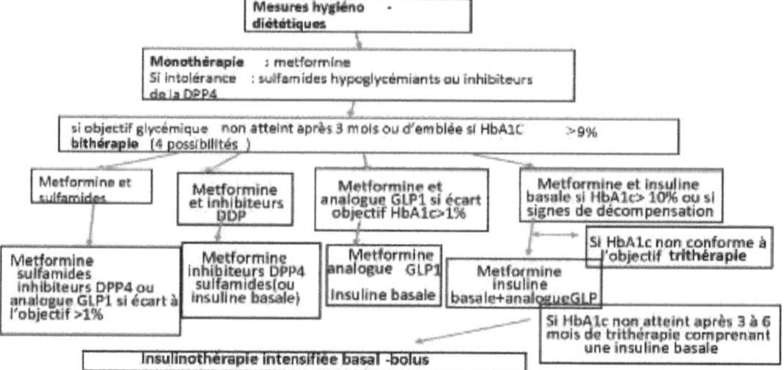

Figure 7 : Medication strategy for glycemic control in type 2 diabetes HAS, 2013

Special cases when diabetes is discovered

> bitherapie d'emblee si HbAlc > 9 % ?

> insulin therapy if HbAlc > 10%, particularly in the presence of symptoms or cephalic bodies.

<u>**Therapeutic strategies defined by the ADA/EASD consensus**</u>

> **Stage 1: monotherapy**
If HbAlc <9%, hygiene and diet measures in combination with metformin

> **Stage 2: bitherapy**
If the objective is not achieved, or if HbAlc > 9%, combine metformin with 1 of the therapeutic classes (hypoglycemic sulphonamides, glitazones, DPP-4 inhibitors, SGLT2 inhibitors, GLP-1 analogues or insulin).

> **Stage 3: tritherapy**
If bitherapy fails
The principle is based on the addition of one of the medicines not yet used.

It is not advisable to combine DPP-4 inhibitors and GLP-1 analogues.

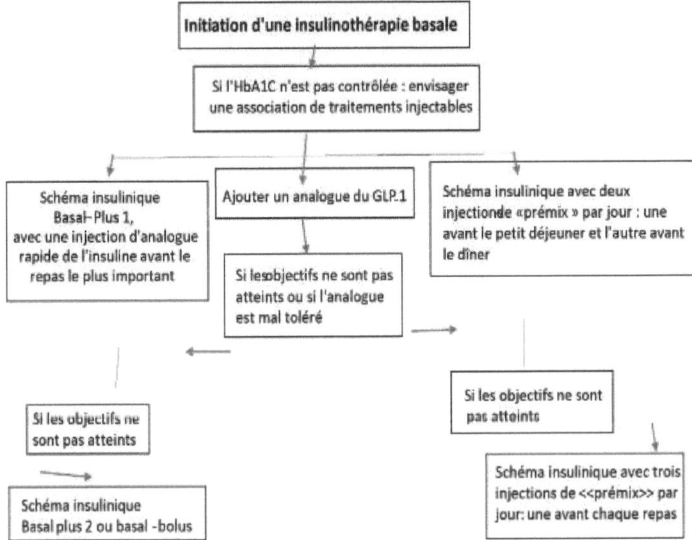

Figure 8: Flowchart recommended by the ADA for combining injectable antidiabetic therapies (insulin and GLP-1 receptor agonists) in type 2 diabetes when HbA1c is not sufficiently controlled or manageable by oral antidiabetics [78].

> Stage 4: insulin therapy

If the target is not achieved after step 3 or if HbA1c >10%, basal insulin therapy should be initiated.
If the objectives are not achieved despite basal insulin therapy, the ADA has defined a therapeutic regimen:
If the objectives are not achieved :
Review insulin treatment plan
1.6.5. Monitoring :

> Insulin diabetes:
Check capillary blood glucose levels before each injection and look for acëtonuria in the event of frank hyperglycëmia;

> Non-insulin treated diabetes:
Optional self-monitoring glycëmique controle glycëmique au moindre proƃlëте.
If you have a disability, a third party will be responsible for supervision:
*   before each insulin injection;
*   once or twice a week in the case of oral treatment.

> Periodic reviews :
Their indication is mainly based on the need for preventive action (particularly secondary and tertiary) to ensure greater comfort.
Scliematiquement :

*** Every 3 months:** HbA1c

The clinical examination will focus mainly on therapeutic evaluation (blood pressure, both horizontal and vertical), weight, nutritional status, general condition, etc.

Table III: Equivalence between HbA1C in % and mean plasma glucose in g/l.

HbA1c	Mean plasma glucose in g/l
4	0,65
5	1,00
6	1,35
7	1,70
8	2,05
9	2,40
10	2,75
11	3,10
12	3,45

*** Once a year :**

ionogram and plasma creatinine (unless an abnormality or associated treatment necessitates closer monitoring); "Complete" urine dipstick Standardised gerontological assessment (see appendices); ECG; ophthalmological examination (fundus, cataract, glaucoma); foot examination: neurological, vascular, deformity and/or abnormal pressure points; Proteinuria.

*** Periodically :**

Carotid ultrasound every 3 years in the absence of warning signs.

2. PARTICULARITIES OF DIABETES IN THE ELDERLY

2.1 Epidemiology :

The over-65s represented 15.8% of the population in 2000, 16.6% in 2010 and are expected to reach 20% by 2020. What's more, as life expectancy increases, the proportion of over-75s is rising sharply. The over-75s currently account for around half of all elderly people, and this proportion is expected to reach 60% in 2050, compared with 53% in 2010. There were around 7 million in 2000, 9 million in 2013 and there will be just over 16 million in 2050 (Blanpain and Buisson, 2016). One of the consequences of these demographic changes is an increase in the prevalence of chronic pathologies (Parker et al. 2014; Prince et al., 2015); there are more and more elderly subjects suffering from several pathologies, and multimorbidity, defined as the coexistence of several chronic pathologies, is increasingly common. In a study conducted in Quebec, where data was collected by general practitioners, subjects aged over 65 had an average of 6 chronic conditions (Fortin et al., 2005).

In 2015, the prevalence of diabetes treated with oral agents or insulin peaked in the 75-79 age group, at almost 21% in men and 15% in women [79]. Its increase was therefore greater than that of the general population, which was 2.1% over the period 2010-2015, and this progression is expected to continue with the increase in life expectancy of the general and diabetic populations, better detection of the disease and, finally, the increase in its incidence Hë mainly due to changes in lifestyle [80].

Often approached as a special case, diabetes in the elderly, due to its increasing frequency and the specificity of the problems it poses, certainly deserves greater attention. There are several difficulties in studying this subject:

2.2 Specificity of diabetes in the elderly [81] :

Can be explained by the combination of :

❖ **Physiological ageing**

- Impaired renal function: measuring creatinine levels is a poor indicator of renal function in the aдë subject. It seems prëfërable to rëfëer to Cockcroft's formula although this is not validëe beyond the age of 80.
- Reduced muscle mass.
- Modification of the pharmacocinUtics of mëdicaments with risk of overdose for water-soluble molUcules and possibility of accumulation and diiTcrcc and prolonдëc action for liposoluble composës.
- Sensory ageing, in particular reduced visual acuity.

❖ **The frequent existence of multiple pathologies**

A source of polymëdication from multiple prescribers, leading to drug interactions. Because of the impact of some of these diseases on quality of life, diseases such as diabetes or hypertension, which are usually asymptomatic, are perceived as minor.

❖ **The heterogeneity of diabetes itself:**

In addition, it should be emphasised that while the vast majority of patients in this age group have type 2 diabetes, the occurrence of long-standing type 1 diabetes is becoming less and less rare [82,83].

In order to provide optimum care for elderly patients, it is necessary to adapt a certain number of requirements to each group of patients, depending on their state of health: **Standardised**

gerontological assessment.

So we can classify them into three(3) categories as follows:

Vigorous older subjects:

They are generally in good health or have a pathology that is correctly treated and well controlled. This case is no longer exceptional but requires a ёvaluation гёдиНёге as these people are likely to slip over the years into one or other of the following categories.

Fragile older people:

They present with several illnesses, nutritional disorders or cognitive impairment. This condition requires careful monitoring to avoid a sudden deterioration into the group of very ill and dependent patients during an acute episode [84].

The definition of frailty is a source of debate in its use in clinical practice. However, **Fried**'s proposal has the merit of simplicity, since a person is considered pre-fragile if they have **2 of 5** criteria and fragile if they have **3. These are** slow walking, weight loss, asthenia, reduced physical activity and muscle weakness [85]. Other valid methods, such as the **SEGA scale** [86], are more competent but take longer to use.

Sick" age subjects:

They are dependent, sometimes at the end of life and often institutionalised. They suffer from a wide range of illnesses requiring numerous treatments, which can lead to iatrogenic accidents. Impairment of cognitive function is particularly common, and these patients are more or less completely dependent on others for everyday activities. The priority therapeutic objectives will be to improve nutritional status and comfort.

2.3 Standardised geriatric assessment :

Numerous studies have shown that it reduces morbidity, mortality and institutionalisation.

Assessment of cognitive functions :

Their integrity determines their ability to carry out everyday tasks.

The Folstein Mini-Mental Test [87] is reliable, valid and easy to administer. It explores memory, learning, mental arithmetic, praxis and gnosis. A score of less than 24/30 should raise suspicions of confusion or dementia and lead to a more precise evaluation. However, the Folstein test is not an early screening test. This assessment of cognitive functions will enable us to adapt or not the education of the diabetic patient and to form an idea of whether or not the patient is complying with treatment.

Assessment of autonomy :

Autonomy corresponds to what the person can actually do in their environment. Here are two validated scales that are easy to use:

-    The ADL (activity of daily living) scale [88, 89], which explores the basic activities of daily living (dressing, washing, etc.);

-    The IADL (instrumental activity of daily living) scale [90] explores the more complex activities of people living at home (shopping, using transport, the telephone, managing one's affairs, etc.).

Assessment of nutritional status :

Malnutrition, which is common in this population, can and does cause significant morbidity: infections, deficiencies, behavioural problems, etc.

The MNA (mini nutritional assessment) [91] is a simple and valid tool.

Assessment of thymic state: depression

Depressive syndromes are common in the elderly with diabetes, but they are often underestimated, especially as they may be confused with early-onset dementia. It is important to be aware of this, especially as appropriate treatment can improve symptoms.

Assessment of the social environment :

It is essential to consider the management of diabetic patients who live at home: close proximity to family, friends, neighbours, home help (nurses, care assistants, physiotherapists, etc.).

2.4 Complications

> Metabolic complications

Hyperosmolar coma is the most frequent form of acute decompensation. In a third of cases, it occurs in the absence of previously known diabetes. The triggering factor of hyperglycemia (severe infection, cerebrovascular accident, myocardial infarction, corticotherapy, massive infusion of glucose solutes, etc.) is frequently associated with a dehydration factor (poor perception of thirst, limited access to water, diuretics, massive sweat or digestive losses) [92].The triggering circumstances should be explained to the patient and those around him, as should the need to ensure correct hydration in any high-risk situation.

Acidocetosis is much rarer in the elderly population where T2DM predominates, and usually reflects the severity of the triggering factor, which frequently determines prognosis [93].

Lactic acidosis almost always results from non-compliance with the rules for using metformin: contraindications linked to renal, hepatic or cardiorespiratory impairment, interruption of treatment in the event of any severe intercurrent pathology with a risk of dehydration.

Hypoglycaemia remains the most feared complication because of its frequency, the difficulty of preventing it and its potential seriousness [94]. Insulin therapy is the most frequent cause, but hypoglycaemic sulphonamides (and repaglinide) also carry a significant risk of severe and prolonged hypoglycaemia [95], particularly when there is an accumulation of the product due to a defect in elimination and/or metabolism (renal or hepatic insufficiency) or a drug-drug interaction concerning in particular the transport or metabolism of the sulphonamide. The symptoms of hypoglycëmia are usually discreet and misleading in aдë subject: dizziness, dësorientation, fall, behavioural disorder of rapid onset.

They can be serious:

+ Through their direct consëquences: dëcompensatıon of vascular or neurological pathology,

+ Through their indirect consëquences: falls, trauma, loss of autonomy, etc. [In the event of rëpëtition, they are likely to affect cognitive functions and may be interpreted as a dëmentiel syndrome.

> Chronic complications

❖ Macroangiopathic complications :

Cardiovascular complications are the cause of dëcës in more than one in two diabetic patients :

Coronary artery disease: [97]

It affects 20% of agëtic diabetics aged 65 to 74 and 28% of those agës over 85. It is frequently not very noisy in terms of its clinical expression and is rëyëк non exceptionally by a complication (myocardial infarction or ECG changes with the appearance of a Q wave, heart failure, sudden death). Coronary angiography is used to confirm the diagnosis and determine the treatment, which should aim to achieve myocardial reperfusion wherever possible. Medical treatment does not differ from that proposed for middle-aged diabetic patients with coronary artery disease.

Heart failure :
Its incidence increases with age [97]. It is doubled in diabetics because of the frequency of hypertension and ischaemic heart disease, but also because of myocardial damage associated with hyperglycaemia. Treatment is based on the same medications as those used in younger patients, but the frequency of associated pathologies and polymedication mean that caution should be exercised when introducing treatments.

Cerebrovascular accident: [98]
It is a major cause of death and serious disability in the elderly. While the risk of hemorrhagic stroke appears to be reduced in diabetics, the risk of ischemic stroke, which sometimes goes unnoticed because of atypical symptoms, is threefold and is increased by the association of hypertension, carotid stenosis or atrial fibrillation. Stroke mortality in diabetics is increased, particularly in the acute phase, by a factor of 1.8 to 3, and both hyperglycaemia and hypoglycaemia appear to be associated with a poorer prognosis. Primary and secondary stroke prevention is based on the same principles as for non-diabetic patients.

Arteriopathy of the lower limbs : [97]
It is a major cause of trophic disorders leading to amputation in elderly diabetics. Because the lesions are so distal and widespread, revascularisation is not always possible. Diagnosis by SPI measurement may be misleading due to mediacalcosis. Medical treatment is not age-specific.

❖ **Micro-angiopathic complications :**
Ophthalmological complications: [97]
Diabetes is the 4th leading cause of blindness in the elderly. Visual problems have a major impact on quality of life and the patient's ability to carry out activities of daily living and manage their treatment. They are a factor in frailty (increased risk of falls, foot sores, etc.) and depression. Loss of vision is due more to edematous maculopathy than to proliferative retinopathy.

Renal complications: [97]
In elderly diabetics, kidney damage is more frequently related to other causes (nephro-angiosclerosis, interstitial nephropathy, obstructive uropathy, etc.) than to diabetic glomerulopathy. Kidney damage is a cause of increased cardiovascular morbidity and mortality and progression to end-stage renal failure. In the event of deterioration in renal function, obstructive uropathy should always be considered, particularly in men, in whom the rectal examination should be systematic.

Neuropathies and trophic disorders of the feet: [97]
All forms of përiphëric, vëgëtative and cranial pair neuropathies ^es to diabëte may be encountered in the адё subject. The associated podiatric risk is increased by foot deformities and difficulties in hygienic care and pëdicuria, favoured by stiffness, visual disorders and paronychia. It is essential to identify patients at particular risk of trophic disorders and to implement preventive measures to limit recourse to amputation with its generally major consequences on the patient's autonomy.

❖ **Other complications**
Apart from cataracts and skin, joint and oral complications [101], which are not particularly specific in elderly subjects, we should mention the relationships between diabetes and various geriatric syndromes [99, 100].

Cognitive disorders :

They are more common in elderly diabetics and should be investigated because of their impact on nutritional status and compliance with treatment. The risk of vascular dementia is doubled in diabetics and multiplied by 6 when associated with hypertension. The link between diabète and Alzheimer's disease, on the other hand, is more debatable. Several observational studies suggest a relationship between poor glycaemic control and impaired cognitive function, as well as a favourable effect of a return to better glycaemic balance.

Depressive states :

Representing a confounding and aggravating factor in a dëmentiel syndrome, they are also more frequent in elderly diabetic patients. They may be exacerbated by the constraints imposed by the treatment of diabetes and the disabilities resulting from its complications. The existence of a depressive syndrome in the elderly diabetic patient is accompanied by an increase in mortality. Its treatment is likely to improve the functional state and therapeutic management of patients.

Nutrition and sarcopenia :

They are powerful determinants of muscle strength and functional capacity, are also more frequent in diabetic patients and may coexist with obesity. These findings should make us particularly vigilant about the risks of low-calorie diets in elderly patients.

Falls and fractures:

The risk is particularly high in patients with long-standing, poorly balanced diabetes, women, people with limited mobility, obese patients or those with orthostatic hypotension, but is probably also increased by hypoglycaemia, peripheral neuropathy, foot deformities, reduced visual acuity and polymedication.

Urinary incontinence :

The risk factors for women with diabetes are the length of time the diabetes has been progressing, neuropathy and obesity, the consequences of which are exacerbated by polyuria resulting from poor glycaemic control.

2.5 Treatment

2.5.1. Specific therapeutic objectives for elderly diabetics

In France, recommendations dating from 2013 recommend adapting the glycemic target to the health status of the elderly subject: the healthier and longer-lived the individual, the stricter the balance should be (HAS 2013). Similar recommendations have been issued in Europe and the United States (Inzucchi et al., 2012). These recommendations suggest adapting the HbA1c target, and consequently the treatment, to the individual's state of health according to the following criteria for the over 75s:

> The so-called "vigorous" elderly, whose life expectancy is considered satisfactory, can benefit from the same targets as younger people, i.e. an HbA1c of less than 7%;

> For the so-called "frail" elderly, an HbAlc target of less than or ёдаle to 8% is recommendёe;

> For so-called 'sick' elderly people, the priority is to avoid acute complications due to hyperglycëmia (dehydration, hyperosmolar coma) and hypoglycëmia; preprandial capillary blood sugars of between 1 and 2 g/l and/or an HbAlc level of less than 9% are recommended. The recommendations issued by the ADA (American Diabetes Association) also recommend that older subjects with no cognitive impairment and a satisfactory life expectancy should

have the same HbAlc targets as younger subjects (Inzucchi et al.,2012). Similarly, the French-speaking Diabeto-gdriatrie group recommends that, from the age of 65, the HbAlc target should be between 6.5 and 7.5% for healthy subjects, and between 7.5 and 8.5% for frail subjects (Alfediam, 2008).

It should be emphasised that while HbA1c targets change according to the state of health of elderly subjects, the drug strategies remain the same.

S **Hygienic-dietetic treatment :**

It still has its place in the elderly. However, as many elderly people prefer carbohydrate foods, it is important to avoid forbidding them to eat foods that could lead to malnutrition or depression. It is essential to know the patient's eating habits so that a balanced eating plan can be drawn up with them, while respecting their tastes. The daily calorie intake should be at least 1,500 calories, and the proposed eating plan should respect the patient's habits. Emphasis is placed on the importance of dividing food intake into at least 3 meals, ensuring an adequate intake of complex carbohydrates, proteins, calcium, iron and vitamins, and the judicious use of high glycemic index sugars at the end of meals.

Physical activity has been shown to be beneficial in the elderly, particularly in terms of muscle trophicity and the risk of falls. It should be recommended for diabetics, but in practice, there are major limitations to the frequency and intensity of physical activity that is likely to have a favourable metabolic and cardiovascular impact. Regular walking should be recommended. More intense activities may be proposed, taking into account the context and after уёпйё 1 the absence of cardiovascular contraindication.

S **Drug treatment**

> **Metformin**

It probably remains an interesting therapeutic agent due to the absence of hypoglycëmic risk and direct drug interaction. In the absence of contraindications, its dosage should not exceed 2g/24 hours in elderly patients. The main limitation to its use is renal insufficiency (GFR [estimated glomerular filtration rate] <60ml/min) due to the risk of lactic acidosis. Other contraindications include severe cardiac and respiratory insufficiency and liver disease.

> **Insulin blockers**

Among the hypoglycaemic sulphonamides, those with a prolonged duration of action (**glipizide** GITS, Gastrointestinal Therapeutic System) are contraindicated in the elderly. **Glibenclamide** should not be used either, as complete elimination of the parent compound and its active metabolites is much slower than predicted from the product's plasma pharmacokinetics, and it is the sulphonamide most frequently implicated in the occurrence of severe hypoglycemia.

> **Repaglinide** may appear to be an attractive alternative due to its rapid elimination, virtually independent of renal function. However, its use is not validated after the age of 75, and there is also a risk of drug interaction, which could lead to severe hypoglycaemia [101].

> **The dipeptidyl peptidase-4 (DP4) inhibitors, sitagliptin, vildagliptin and saxagliptin**, offer the advantage of good tolerability and no risk of hypoglycaemia when combined with an insulin-sensitising agent. The results of studies have led most expert groups to recommend them as second-line therapy after metformin in elderly diabetics [99-101, 102].

However, the benefits of **GLP-1 analogues, exenatide and liraglutide,** in combination with metformin + hypoglycaemic sulphonamide or insulin, have not been established in *elderly* *patients. In* addition to their action on rinsulinosecretion, *these* agents slow gastric emptying and have a satietogenic effect which may be detrimental in subjects who are more prone to malnutrition.

> Alphaglucosidase inhibitors (acarbose, miglitol)

They may appear attractive due to their lack of systemic effects. However, their often poor digestive tolerance and limited efficacy mean that they are usually only an adjunctive therapeutic class [101].

> Sodium-glucose cotransporter (SGLT2) inhibitors or gliflozins

It appears promising in terms of preventing cardiac complications (particularly heart failure) and renal failure, and reducing mortality. However, experience is limited in elderly patients, and the risk of malnutrition due to urinary glucose leakage, dehydration and hypotension suggest caution in frail patients [99].

> Insulin therapy

It often appears to be the best therapeutic approach, whether for patients with long-standing, polymedic diabetes, or where there are contraindications to the use of oral agents. It undoubtedly has a favourable impact on the quality of life of patients who were previously chronically unbalanced. Therapeutic regimens should be adapted [99, 101] and monitoring (education of the patient and those around him) should be introduced to minimise the risk of hypoglycaemia, which can have harmful effects when it occurs in a patient with diffuse vascular disease. All the therapeutic regimens used in young people can be offered to independent elderly patients. Simple regimens such as twice-daily injections of an NPH or Premix insulin are often preferred for frail or dependent patients whose treatment is managed by a family member or home nurse.

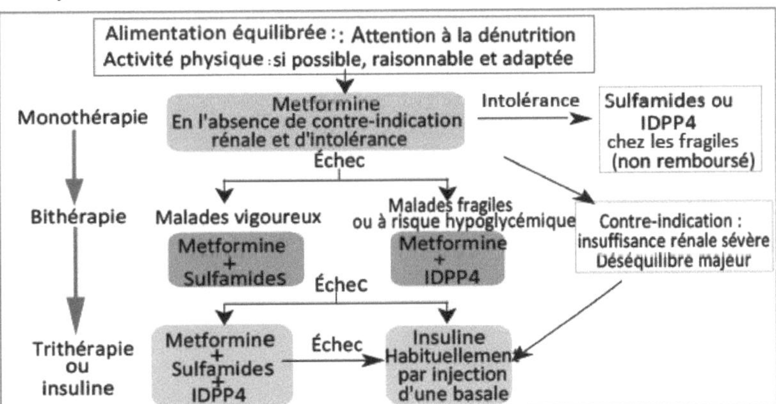

Figure 9: Therapeutic strategy [103]

2.5.2. Monitoring and therapeutic education of elderly diabetics

The ENTRED 2007 study [104] confirms that coronary, ophthalmological and podiatric complications increase with age in older subjects, but contrary to what some older studies suggest, it does not reveal any major differences in the distribution of HbA1c, blood pressure and lipid levels between the different age groups up to the age of 80. This means that older diabetic patients should be monitored in the same way as younger patients, or even more closely, given the frequency of associated cardiac, ophthalmological or renal pathologies not directly related to diabetes. The most specific aspects of monitoring elderly patients involve regularly updating the list of treatments prescribed by various healthcare professionals, identifying possible drug interactions and checking compliance with treatment.

Table IV: Monitoring of elderly diabetics in situations other than those requiring reinforced controls **(based on [105]).**

Monitoring	Features
Daily	- Glycemic self-monitoring in the case of insulin treatment : • adapted to the therapeutic plan • reinforced in the event of intercurrent disease - carried out by a third party in the event of loss of independence - Adapting doses according to a written protocol - Optional self-monitoring in the case of oral treatment
Quarterly	- Clinical examination: weight, nutritional status, hydration, supine and standing BP - HbA1c
Annual	- Oral and dental examination - Cardiovascular: ECG - Feet: sensitivity, pulse, deformities, skin problems - Gerontological assessment - Creatinine, plasma ionogram, microalbuminuria or proteinuria, urine dipstick - Lipid profile - Ophthalmological examination
Every 3 years	- Dopplers of the supraaortic trunks and the axes of the lower limbs should be performed even in the absence of symptoms.

3 METHODOLOGY :

3.1 Setting and location of the study:

This was a тепёе study in the internal medicine department of the Centre Hospitalier Mёre-Enfant (CHME) le Luxembourg in the city of Bamako which includes:

-Administration ;

-Medical departments: internal medicine, cardiology, nephrology, paediatrics, oncology, etc.

-Surgical departments: general surgery, intensive care and emergency medicine, obstetric gynaecology,

-A medical imaging department, an analysis laboratory and a hospital pharmacy.

3.2 Type and period of study :

This was a descriptive cross-sectional study with prospective data collection, from 01 July 2020 to 31 December 2020 (six (6) months).

3.3 Study population :

Our study was conducted on subjects aged 65 and over, who had an inpatient stay in the internal medicine department of the Mёre-Enfant CHME "LE LUXEMBOURG" hospital centre.

3.4 Sample size and sampling

As the sampling is exhaustive, the sample size N cannot be calculated:

3.5 Inclusion criteria :

Our study included all subjects aged 65 or over with diabetes who had been hospitalised at our study site during the study period, had a usable record and consented to take part in the study.

3.6 Non-inclusion criteria :

Our study did not include any elderly diabetic subjects who refused to take part in the study and/or whose files were incomplete.

3.7 Data collection phase :

Data were collected on an individual, pre-prepared survey form addressed to elderly diabetic patients hospitalised during the study period. The questionnaire was tested and validated before use in the study.

3.8 Variables

•   Sociodёmographic variables: surname, first name(s), age, sex, BMI, питёго identifier, ethnicity, place of residence ;

•   Clinical variables :

-   Antёcёdents: personal and family;

-   Diabёte and cardiovascular risk factors: modifiable and non-modifiable

-   History of diabёte: Date of dёcouverte, mode of dёcouverte, type of diabёte, follow-up, acute, chronic, podological and infectious complications, initial and current treatment; search for secondary causes of diabёte.

-   Hospitalisation data: reason for admission, examination дёпёга!, physical examination, complete blood count (CBC, HBA1C, lipidogram, blood ionogram, TSHus, Creati^mia, microalbuminuria, lipasemia, troponins, pancreatic area X-ray, chest X-ray, ECBU, ECG, Echocoeur), treatment.

- Variables gёronte-gёriatriques :   : Mini mental Score (MMS), Mini Nutritional Assessment (MNS), Mobile and risk of falling (Up & GO test), Activities of Daily Living, mini-Geriatric Depression Scale.

3.9 Operational definitions :

- Polymëdication: This is defined as the simultaneous administration of numerous drugs or the administration of an excessive number of drugs. The threshold of drugs set by the WHO is 5 or more.

- A hemoglobin level of <13g/dl in men and <12g/dl in women was considered anemia.

- A leucocyte count greater than 10,000/::-::-r was considered hyperleucocytosis.

- **University of Texas classification**

	9 Grade O Epithelial lesion	Grade 1 Superficial wound	I Grade 2 Tendon or capsule damage	Grade 3i Bone or joint damage
Stage A No infection No ischemia	OA (O %)	1A (O %)	2A (O %)	SA (O %)
Stage B infection No ischemia	OB (12.5%)	1 B (8,5 %)	2B (28,6 %)	SB (92%)
Stage C No infection Ischemie	OC (25%)	1 C (20 %)	2C (25 %)	SC (1 OO %)
Stage D Infection and ischemia	OD (50%)	1 D (50 %)	2D (100 %)	3D (100 %)

- **Glycemic balance in the elderly:**

- The so-called "vigorous" elderly: HbAlc less than 7%;

- For the so-called "frail" elderly, an HbAlc target of less than or ёдale to 8% is recommended;

- For "sick" elderly people: HbA1c of less than 9% is recommended.

- Body mass index (BMI) :

BMI <21: malnutrition or starvation; 21< BMI>24.99: normal;

BMI> 25: Overweight;   30<BMI>34,99 : ObesitemodSree   ;

35<BMI>40 :Severe obesity; BMI>40 : Morbid obesity

-A total score of 30 reassures the patient

MMS :   - Between 20 and 30, the diagnosis cannot be made.

- Below 20, there is a real problem

- **UP& GO:** risk of falling if score < 1 and completion time > 20 seconds.

Slow execution, hesitation and a very shaky pace were also noticeable.

- **IADL:** 0 designating total dysautonomia and 8 a totally autonomous person

- **MMA:** Normal if score > 12; If score <11 malnutrition likely

- **GDS > 1**, the probability of depression is high (sensitivity: 88%, specificity: 63%)

3.10 Data analysis :

The data were processed and analysed using SPSS version 21 software and the results will be presented in the form of text, tables and graphs using Word office version 2013 software. We used P<0.05 as the significance level for the statistical tests in order to compare the different results.

3.11 Ethical considerations :

A free and clear consent was obtained from each patient or their guardian before inclusion in our study. Refusal by the patient or his or her guardian to participate in our study in no way hindered the proper management of the patient in the department or elsewhere. All information given by the patient was completely confidential, and the anonymity of our patients was preserved by assigning to each patient a number that did not allow the patient to be identified during the investigation or publication of our work.j

43

4 RESULTS

4.1 Overall results :

During our study period, 254 patients were hospitalised, including 38 elderly diabetic subjects, representing a **hospital frequency** of **14.96%.** Of these 38 diabetic patients 30 met our inclusion criteria, i.e. **11.81%.**

4.2 Descriptive results :

S **Socio-demographic data :**

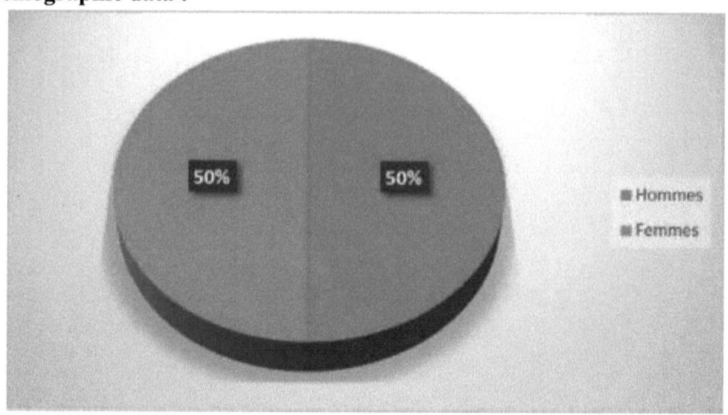

Figure 10: Breakdown by gender

Men and women each represented 50% of the total workforce, giving a sex ratio of 1.

Table V: Age distribution

Age groups	Workforce	Percentage
65-74 years	**17**	**56,7**
75-84 years	9	30,0
85-95 years	4	13,3
Total	30	100,0

The 65-74 age group accounted for 56.7%. The mean age was 75.23±7.29. The extremes were 65 and 90 years.

Table VI: Distribution by ethnic group

Ethnic group	Workforce	Percentage
Bambara	**11**	**36,7**
Malinke	7	23,3
Sarakole	5	16,7
Peulh	3	10,0
Bozo	1	3,3
Wolof	1	3,3
Mianka	1	3,3
Diawando	1	3,3
Total	30	100,0

The Bambara ethnic group accounted for 36.7% of cases.

Table VII: Breakdown by occupation

Profession	Workforce	Percentage
Housewife	**12**	**40,0**
Teacher	8	26,7
Worker	4	13,3
Uniform carrier	2	6,7
Health agent	1	3,3
Agent for rural development	1	3,3
Berger	1	3,3
Retailer	1	3,3
Total	30	100,0

Housewives accounted for 40% of cases.

S **Clinical data:**

> **Reason for hospitalisation:**

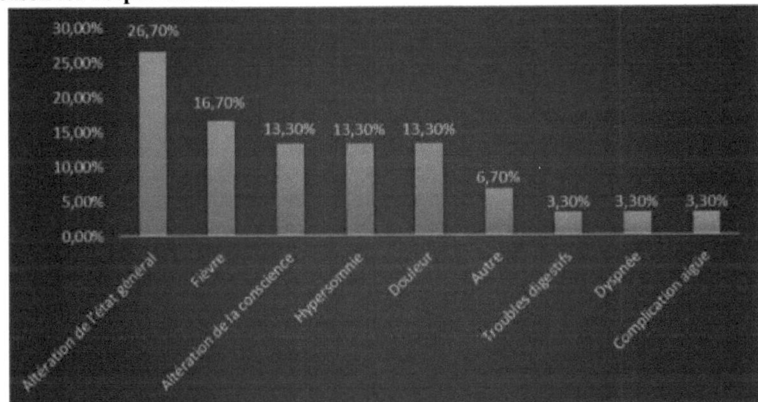

Figure 11 : Breakdown by reason for hospitalisation **Altered general condition** accounted for 26.7% of cases.

> **Antecedents and cardiovascular risk factors:**

Tableau VIII Breakdown by personal background

Personal history	Number N=30	Percentage
Arterial hypertension	**25**	**83,3**
Osteoarthritis	16	53,3
Dyslipidemia	11	36,6
Overweight or obese	6	20,0
Hepatopathy	4	13,3
Gastroraphy	2	6,6
Heart disease (undocumented)	2	6,6
Rheumatoid arthritis	1	3,3
No	1	3,3

Arterial hypertension was present in 83.3% of cases.

Tableau IX Breakdown by family background

Family background	Number N=30	Percentage
Meconnus	**18**	**60,0**
Arterial hypertension	**9**	**30,0**
Diabdte	7	23,3
Drepanocytosis	4	13,3
Heart disease	3	10,0
Epilepsy	1	3,3
Chronic psychosis	1	3,3
Asthma	1	3,3

Arterial hypertension was found as a family antecedent in 30% of cases; 60% of our patients had no known family antdcddent.

Tableau X   : Breakdown by BMI

Body Mass Index	Workforce	Percentage
Normal	8	26,7
Overweight	**11**	**36,7**
Moderate obesity	6	20,0
Severe obesity	3	10,0
Morbid obesity	2	6,7
Total	30	100,0

The majority of our patients (36.7%) were overweight, and only 26.7% had a normal BMI.

Tableau XI Breakdown by lipid profile

Dyslipidemia	Workforce	Percentage
Yes	**21**	**70,0**
No	9	30,0
Total	30	100,0

Dyslipidemia was present in 70% of cases.

Table XII: Breakdown according to whether the patient is sedentary or not

sëdentaritë	Workforce	Percentage
Yes	16	53,3
No	14	46,7
Total	30	100,0

The sëdentaritë ёlак. гейоиуёе in 53.3% of cases.

> **History of diabetes :**

Table XIII: Rëpartition by duration of diabetes progression.

How long does diabetes progress?	Workforce	Percentage
Less than 10 years old	13	43,3

Between 10 and 20 years	**16**	**53,3**
Over 20 years	1	3,3
Total	30	100,0

The duration of diabetes progression was between 10 and 20 years, representing 53.3%.

Table XIV: Breakdown by type of diabetes diagnosis

How diabetes is discovered	Workforce	Percentage
Assessment of a polyuro-polydipsic syndrome	**26**	**86,7**
Acute cëto-acidosis complication	2	6,7
Chronic complication	2	6,7
Total	30	100,0

The mode of dëcouverte ëtait syndrome polyuro-polydipsic in 86.7% of cases.

Table XV: Breakdown by type of diabetes

Type of diabetes	Workforce	Percentage
Type 1	0	0,0%
Type2	30	100,0
Secondary diabetes	0	0,0%

Type 2 diabetes accounted for 100% of cases.

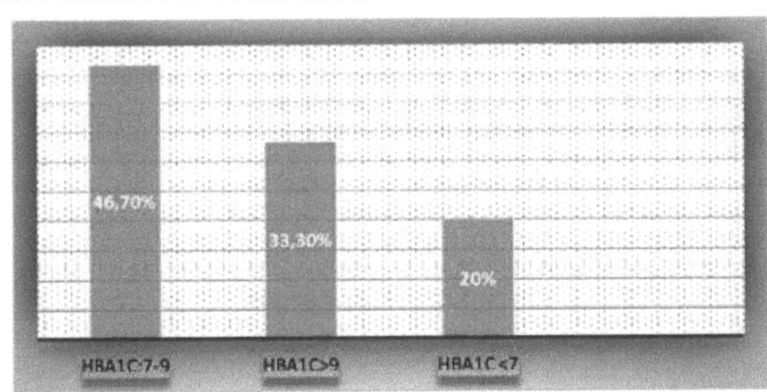

Figure 12: Distribution according to glycemic balance

I . The glycaemoglobin of our patients was between 7% and 9% in 46.7% of cases.

Table XVI: Breakdown by acute complications of diabetes

Acute complications	Workforce	Percentage
Hyperosmolarity	2	6,7
Cetoacidosis	**4**	**13,3**
Hypoglycemia	**4**	**13,3**
No	20	66,7
Total	30	100,0

Acute complications were dominated by hypoglycaemia and cetoacidosis, accounting for 13.3% each.

Table XVII: Breakdown by chronic microangiopathic complications of diabetes

Microangiopathic complications	Number N=30	Percentage
Retinopathy	6	20,0
Neuropathy	**9**	**30,0**
Retinopathy +Nephropathy	1	3,3
Retinopathy + Neuropathy	4	13,3
Retinopathy+Nephropathy+Neuropathy	3	10,0
No	7	23,3

Neuropathy was the microangiopathic complication in 53.33% of cases.

Table XVIII: Breakdown by chronic macoangiopathic complications of diabetes

Macoangiopathic complications	Number N=30	Percentage
Ischemic heart disease	1	3,3
AOMI	1	3,3
HTA	**15**	**50,0**
Ischemic heart disease + AOMI	1	3,3
HTA+AVC	6	20,0
Hypertension+OAD+Ischemic heart disease	1	3,3
Hypertension+Stroke+Ischemic heart disease	2	6,7
HTA+AOMI	1	3,3
No	2	6,7

Arterial hypertension was found in 83.33% of cases.

Table XIX: Breakdown by acute infectious complications

Site of infectious complications	Number N=30	Percentage
Pulmonary	**14**	**46,6**
Digestive tract	1	3,3
Cutane	5	16,6
Uro-genital	2	6,6
No	10	33,3

Infectious complications (pulmonary, digestive, cutaneous and urogenital) were present in 66.6% of our patients. Pulmonary infection alone accounted for 46.6% of cases.

Table XX: Distribution according to the Texas classification

Texas classification (Stage/Grade)	Workforce	Percentage
No wound	**25**	**83,3**
A0	**2**	**6,7**
B2	**1**	**3,3**
D3	**1**	**3,3**

| B1 | 1 | 3,3 |
| Total | 30 | 100,0 |

Class A0 was the most common, representing 6.7% of cases.

***f* Overall geriatric assessment data**

Table XXI: Breakdown by patient cognition

Cognitive impairment(MMS)	Workforce	Percentage
No	**15**	**50,0**
Vascular dementia	**9**	**30,0**
Alzheimer's disease	6	20,0
Total	30	100,0

The тоШё of our patients had no cognitive impairment and of the remainder patients with vascular dementia accounted for 60%.

Table XXII: Rëpartition according to paticnt autonomy

Autonomy (ADL/IADL)	Workforce	Percentage
Yes	**17**	**56,7**
No	13	43,3
Total	30	100,0

Independent patients accounted for 56.7%.

Table XXIII: Rëpartition by nutritional status of patients.

Malnutrition (MNA)	Workforce	Percentage
No	**21**	**70,0**
Yes	9	30,0
Total	30	100,0

Undernutrition was found in 30% of cases.

Table XXIV: Distribution of patients according to their thymic state

Depression(MGSD)	Workforce	Percentage
No	**23**	**76,7**
Yes	7	23,3
Total	30	100,0

Depression was present in 23.3% of patients.

Table XXV: Distribution of patients according to their risk of falling

Risk of falling (Up& Go test)	Workforce	Percentage
Yes	**17**	**56,7**
No	13	43,3
Total	30	100,0

Patients at risk of falling accounted for 56.7%.

Table XXVI: Breakdown by medication

Polymedication	Workforce	Percentage
Yes	**20**	**66,7**
No	10	33,3
Total	30	100,0

Polymecation was found in 66.7% of patients.

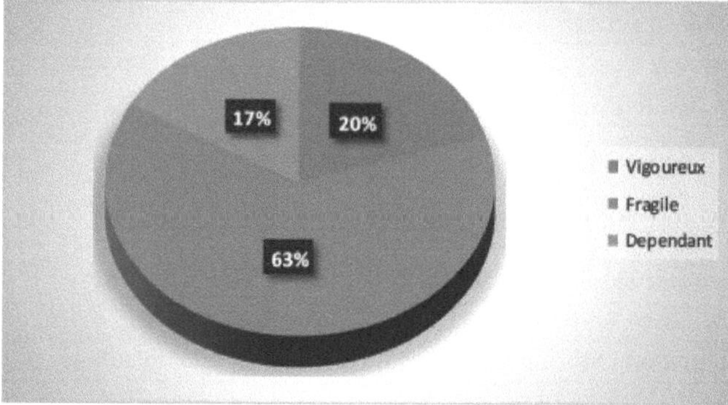

Figure 13: Breakdown by overall geriatric assessment of patients

Frail patients accounted for 63%.

S **Paraclinical tests**

Table XXVII : Distribution according to the presence or absence of **Dysthyroidism**

Dysthyroidism	Workforce	Percentage
No	**28**	**93,3**
Yes	2	6,7
Total	30	100,0

Dysthyroidism was present in 6.7% of cases.

Table XXVIII : Distribution according to hemoglobin level

Anemie	Workforce	Percentage
No	**19**	**63,3**
Yes	11	36,7
Total	30	100,0

anemia was found in 36.7% of cases.

Table XXIX: Distribution according to the presence or absence of neutrophil hyperleukocytosis

Neutrophil hyperleukocytosis	Workforce	Percentage
Yes	**16**	**53,3**
No	14	46,7
Total	30	100,0

Neutrophil hyperleukocytosis was present in 53.3% of our patients.

S **Therapeutic aspects**

> Treatment of diabetes

Table XXX: Distribution of patients according to whether or not they were prescribed treatment at the time of discovery of diabetes

Treatment since discovery	Workforce	Percentage
Yes	**29**	**96,7**
No	1	3,3
Total	30	100,0

Ninety-six point seven percent (96.7%) of our patients were treated from the time of discovery.

Tableau XXXI   Breakdown by initial diabetes treatment

Initial treatment	Number N=30	Percentage
Oral antidiabetic	**15**	**50,0**
Insulin	10	33,3
Regime	4	13,3
Oral antidiabetic and Insulin	1	3,3

Half of our patients were initially on oral antidiabetics.

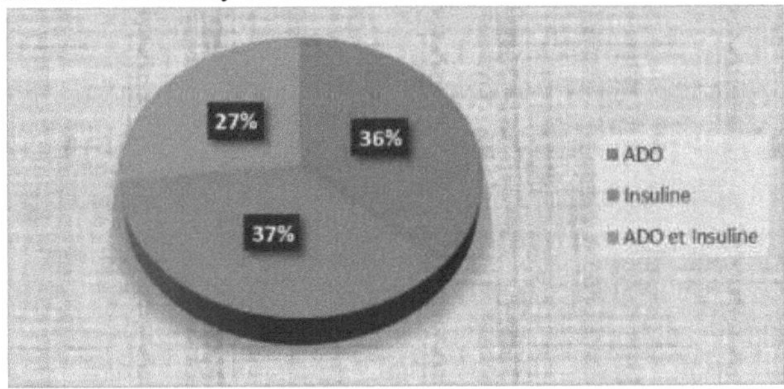

Figure 14: Distribution according to current diabetes treatment

Insulin-only patients were the most represented, at 37%.

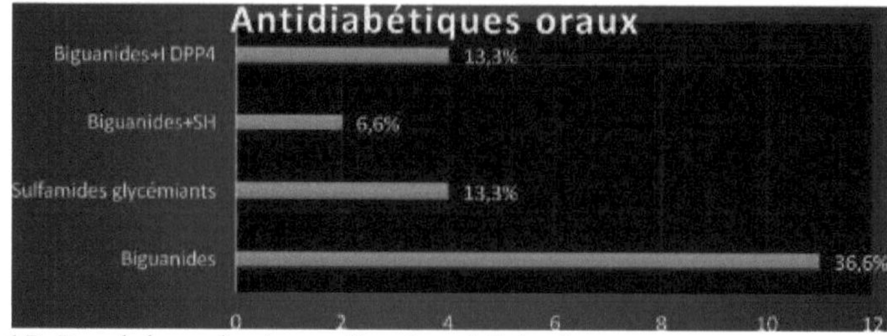

Figure 15: Breakdown by type of oral antidiabetic agent

Metformin (Biguanide), prescribed alone or in combination with other OADs, had a frequency of use of 56.6%.

> **Treatment of co-morbidities**

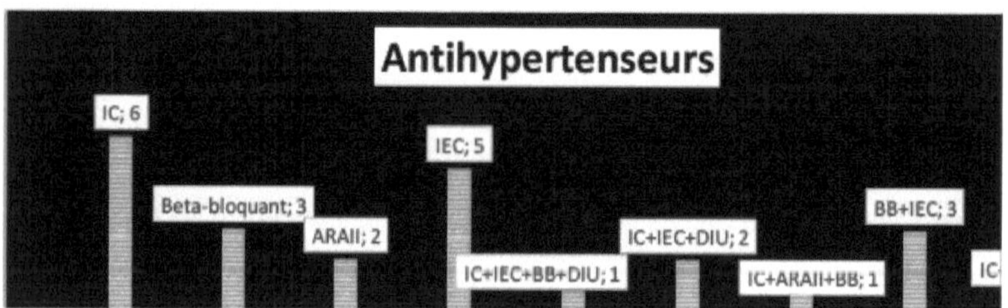

Figure 16: Breakdown by type of antihypertensive drug

Calcium ё inhibitors were ийНзёз in 36.6% of cases.

Tableau XXXII   : Rёpartition by type of treatment ЬуроНрётхаП;

Lipid-lowering treatment	Workforce	Percentage
Statins	14	46,7
Fibrates	1	3,3
No	15	50,0
Total	30	100,0

The lipid-lowering treatment ё1:ш1: a statin in 46.7% of cases.

Tableau XXXIII Distribution according to whether or not **platelet anti-aggregants are** taken

Antiplatelet agents	Workforce	Percentage
Yes	**22**	**73,3**
No	8	26,7
Total	30	100,0

Patients on anti-platelet agents accounted for 73.3%.

4.3 Analytical results

TableXXXIV : **Relationship between patients' glycaemoglobin and age**

Age	Hbalc			Total

	Hba1c<7%	Hba1c:7%-9%		Hba1c >9%			
	np%	n	p%	n	p%	N	P%
65-74 years	529,4	4	23,5	8	47,1	17	100,0
75-84 years	00,0	8	88,9	1	11,1	9	100,0
85-95 years	125,0	2	50,0	1	25,0	4	100,0
Total	620,0	14	46,7	10	33,3	30	100,0

We foundë a statically significant association between HBA1c and age; **P =0.035.**
The majority of patients aged between 65 and 74 years had a Hbalc > 9% (n=8), i.e. 47.1%.
The majority of patients aged 75-84 years had an Hbalc of between 7% and 9% (n=8), i.e. 88.9%, as did patients aged 85-95 years (n=2), i.e. 50%.

Table XXXV: Patients' glycemic hemoglobin according to their overall geriatric assessment

overall geriatric assessment	Hbalc					Total	
	Hbalc<7%		Hbalc:7%-9%		IIbalc >9%		
	n	p%	n	p%	n	p%	N	P%
vigorous	5	83,3	1	16,7	0	0,0	6	100,0
Fragile	1	5,3	9	47,7	9	47,7	19	100,0
Dependant	0	0,0	4	80,0	1	20,0	5	100,0
Total	6	20,0	14	46,7	10	33,3	30	100,0

We found a statistically significant association between gëriatric re-evaluation and HBA1c **P=0.00.**

The majority of vigorous patients had an Hbalc <7% (n=5), i.e. 83.3%; only 5.3% (n=1) of frail patients had an Hbalc <7% (n=5), while the majority of dependent patients had an Hbalc between 7% and 9% (n=4), i.e. 80%.

Table XXXVI: Patients' glycemic balance and the occurrence of microangiopathic complications of diabetes

Micoangiopathies	Hbalc						Total	
	Hbalc<7%		Hbalc:7%-9%		Hbalc >9%			
	n	p%	n	p%	n	p%	N	P%
Retinopathy	0	0,0	2	33,3	4	66,7	6	100,0
Neuropathy	1	11,1	5	55,6	3	33,3	9	100,0
Retinopathy+Nephropathy	0	0,0	1	100,0	0	0,0	1	100,0
Retinopathy+neuropathy	1	25,0	3	75,0	0	0,0	4	100,0
Retinopathy+Nephropathy+Neuropathy	0	0,0	2	66,7	1	33,3	3	100,0
No	4	57,1	1	14,2	2	28,6	7	100,0
Total	6	20,0	14	46,7	10	33,3	30	100,0

We found no statistical association between glycemic imbalance and the occurrence of microangiopathic complications; **P=0.1.**

Table XXXVII: **Patients' glycemic balance and the occurrence of macoangiopathic complications** of diabetes

Macroangiopathies	Hba1c						Total	
	Hba1c<7%		Hba1c:7% 9		Hba1c >9%			
	n	p%	n	p%	n	p%	N	P%
Ischemic heart disease	1	100,0	0	0,0	0	0,0	1	100,0
AOMI	0	0,0	1	100,0	0	0,0	1	100,0
HTA	3	20,0	6	40,0	6	40,0	15	100,0
HTA+AOMI	0	0,0	1	100,0	0	0,0	1	100,0
Heart disease I+ AOMI	0	0,0	0	0,0	1	100,0	1	100,0
HTA+AVC	1	16,6	4	66,7	1	16,6	6	100,0
High blood pressure + OSA + Heart disease I	0	0,0	1	100,0	0	0,0	1	100,0
High blood pressure + stroke + heart disease I	0	0,0	1	50,0	1	50,0	2	100,0
No	1	50,0	0	0,0	1	50,0	2	100,0
Total	6	20,0	14	46,7	10	33,3	30	100,0

Heart disease I: Ischaemic heart disease

We did not find a statistical association between glycaemic imbalance and the occurrence of macroangiopathic complications; **P=0.6.**

Table XXXVIII: Occurrence of microangiopathic complications of diabetes as a function of age

Microangiopathic complications	Age						Total	
	65-74 years		75-84 years		85-95 years			
	n	p%	n	p%	n	p%	N	P%
Retinopathy	3	50,0	2	33,3	1	16,7	6	100,0
Neuropathy	7	77,7	1	11,1	1	11,1	9	100,0
Retinopathy+Nephropathy	0	0,0	1	100,0	0	0,0	1	100,0
Retinopathy+neuropathy	1	25,0	2	50,0	1	25,0	4	100,0
Retinopathy+Nephropathy+Neuropathy	2	66,7	1	33,3	0	0,0	3	100,0
No	4	57,1	2	28,5	1	14,2	7	100,0
Total	17	56,7	9	30,0	4	13,3	30	100,0

We found no statistically significant association between advancing age and the occurrence of microangiopathic complications; **P=0.7.**

Table XXXIX: Occurrence of macroangiopathic complications of diabetes as a function of age

Macroangiopathic complications	Age						Total	
	65-74 years		75-84 years		85-95 years			
	n	p%	n	p%	n	p%	N	P%
Ischemic heart disease	1	100,0	0	0,0	0	0,0	1	100,0
AOMI	1	100,0	0	0,0	0	0,0	1	100,0
HTA	8	53,3	5	33,3	2	13,3	15	100,0
HTA+AOMI	1	100,0	0	0,0	0	0,0	1	100,0
Heart disease I+ AOMI	1	100,0	0	0,0	0	0,0	1	100,0

	n	p%	n	p%	n	p%	N	P%
HTA+AVC	3	50,0	3	50,0	0	0,0	6	100,0
High blood pressure + OSA + Heart disease I	0	0,0	0	0,0	1	100,0	1	100,0
High blood pressure + stroke + heart disease I	1	50,0	1	50,0	0	0,0	2	100,0
No	1	50,0	0	0,0	1	50,0	2	100,0
Total	17	56,7	9	30,0	4	13,3	30	100,0

We found no statistically significant association between advancing age and the occurrence of macroangiopathic complications; **P=0.5.**

Table XL: Occurrence of acute complications' of diabetes according to overall gerontological assessment

Acute complications s'	Global geriatric assessment						Total	
	Vigorous		Fragile p%		Dependant			
	n	p%	n		n	p%	N	P%
Hyperosmolarity	1	50,0	1	50,0	0	0,0	2	100,0
Cdto-acidosis	0	0,0	4	100,0	0	0,0	4	100,0
Hypoglycemia	1	25,0	1	25,0	2	50,0	4	100,0
No	4	20,0	13	65,0	3	15,0	20	100,0
Total	6	20,0	19	63,3	5	16,7	30	100,0

We did not find a statistically significant association between the state of our patients according to global geriatric assessment and the occurrence of acute complications; **P=0.8.**

Table XLI: Occurrence of microangiopathic complications according to overall gerontological assessment

Microangiopathic complications	Global geriatric assessment						Total	
	Vigorous		Fragile		Dependan			
	n	p%	n	p%	n	p%t	N	P%
Retinopathy	0	0,0	6	100,0	0	0,0	6	100,0
Neuropathy	1	11,1	8	88,9	0	0,0	9	100,0
Retinopathy+ Nephropathy	0	0,0	0	0,0	1	100,0	1	100,0
Retinopathy+ Neuropathy	0	0,0	2	50,0	2	50,0	4	100,0
Retinopathy+Nephropathy+Neuropathy	0	0,0	2	75,0	1	25,0	3	100,0
No	5	71,4	1	14,3	1	14,3	7	100,0
Total	6	20,0	19	63,3	5	16,3	30	100,0

We found a statistically significant association between overall geriatric assessment and the occurrence of microangiopathic complications. **P= 0,02.**

The vigorous elderly subjects were predominantly free of microangiopathic complications (n=5), i.e. 71.4%, whereas the frail elderly subjects were predominantly affected by neuropathy (n=8), i.e. 88.9%, and the dependent patients were predominantly affected by retinopathy associated with neuropathy(2), i.e. 50%.

TableXLII: Distribution of macroangiopathic complications according to overall geriatric assessment

Macroangiopathic complications	Global geriatric assessment						Total	
			Fragile		Dependant			
	n	Vigorous p%	n	p%	n	p%	N	P%
Ischemic heart disease	1	100,0	0	0,0	0	0,0	1	100,0
AOMI	0	0,0	1	100,0	0	0,0	1	100,0
HTA	3	20,0	11	73,3	1	6,7	15	100,0
HTA+AOMI	0	0,0	1	100,0	0	0,0	1	100,0
Heart disease I+ AOMI	0	0,0	1	100,0	0	0,0	1	100,0
HTA+AVC	1	16,6	4	66,7	1	16,6	6	100,0
High blood pressure + OSA + Heart disease I	0	0,0	0	0,0	1	100,0	1	100,0
High blood pressure + stroke + heart disease I	0	0,0	1	50,0	1	50,0	2	100,0
No	1	50,0	0	0,0	1	50,0	2	100,0
Total	6	20,0	19	63,3	5	16,7	30	100,0

We found no statistically significant association between the condition of our patients and the occurrence of macroangiopathy; **P=0.3.**

Table XLIII: Breakdown by geriatric status of patients and number of medicines taken by the patient.

Global geriatric assessment	Polymedication				Total	
	Yes		No			
	n	p%	n	p%	N	P%
vigorous	1	16,7	5	83,3	6	100,0
fragile	14	73,7	5	26,3	19	100,0
dependent	5	100,0	0	0,0	5	100,0
Total	20	66,7	10	33,3	30	100,0

We found a statistically significant association between polymëdication and the state of

our patients has Overall gëriatric evaluation; **P=0.008.**

Only 16.7% (n=1) of the vigorous patients ëtait polymëdiquës; the frail patients ëtait mostly polymëdiquës (n=14), i.e. 73.4%; the ^'be^ë of our dëpendent patients ëtait polymëdiquë (n=5), i.e. 100%.

5 COMMENTS AND DISCUSSION

5.1 Limitations of the study :

• The socio-economic conditions in dëfavorables meant that many of our patients were unable to undergo certain tests to check for chronic complications.

• The dëcës of certain patients prior to the completion of their overall gëriatric ë assessment, which ëwas the cause of their non-inclusion in the study.

• the small size of our ë^^ИЬ^

5.2 Frequency :

At the end of our ëШëc, we found a hospital frequency of 14.96%. This result is lower than that found by Dienta F (22.61%) in 2009 [106] and that found in a similar study in the internal medicine department of Point G (27.73%). This could be explained by the small size of our ëample, the divergence between our përiods of study and the fact that Point G had ëtë during this përiod a rëfërence in diabetes management.

5.3 Socio-demographic aspects

Gender:

In our ëШëc, 15 patients ëtaient de sexe fëminin et 15 de sexe masculin, soit un sexe ratio de 1. Ceci ëtait proche de celui trouvë par Mahamane Sani et al au Niger en 2018 et J ABODO et al qui retrouvës respectivement 1,24% et 0,97% [107,108]. On the other hand, according to the 2019 statistics provided by the IDF, the prevalence of diabëte is more ëlevëe in men

Age :

The mean age ëtait 75.23 years with extremes ranging from 65 to 90 years. This result was slightly more ëkyë than that of Mahamane Sani et al which was 70 years [107], similar to those found by Sophie B and M.-A. Chami et al which were 76.7 ± 5.9 years [109] and 75.9 [110] respectively.

5.4 Clinical aspects :

Reason for hospitalisation :

The ah^ration de l'état gënëral (AEG), a fairly frequent mode of discovery of a pathology, was the most common reason for hospitalisation in our study, at 26.7%. This result was higher than that of C. GEIST in 2013 in the Strasbourg emergency department, which had a frequency of 21% [111]. This could be explained by the fact that AEG is an infrequent reason for hospitalisation in emergency departments compared with other reasons, unlike internal medicine.

Hypoglycëmia is nevertheless cited in the literature as ëbeing the most frequent.

Type of diabetes :

Type 2 diabetes was the type of diabëte found in all our patients (100%). We did not record any secondary diabëte. Dienta F [106] and M.-A. Chami et al [110] found a similar result, i.e. 100%. Mahamane Sani et al and J.ABODO et al found approximately the same result, i.e. 93.3% and 96.2% respectively [107,108]. This can be explained by the fact that type 2 diabëte represents the major part of diabëtes, as stated in the literature.

The two (2) dysthyroidies (hypothyroidism) found during the study were discovered during the course of diabëte resolution, and none of the patients had undergone an abdominal X-ray to look for calcification in the pancreatic air. The aim of these additional examinations was to search for a secondary cause of the diabetes.

Modifiable and non-modifiable diabetes and cardiovascular risk factors :

Given their age (65 or over), all our patients already had at least one non-modifiable diabetes and cardiovascular risk factor. The presence of at least one modifiable risk factor for diabetes was found in 86.7%.

Sedentary lifestyle was present in 53.3% of our patients. M.-A. Chami et al found a frequency of 57% [110], J.ABODO et al, 57.4% [108] and Mahamane Sani et al, a frequency of 85.6% [107].

Overweight was present in 36.7% of cases. This result was similar to that found by Dienta F (36.58%) [106], close to those found by MA. Chami et al and K Diyane et al, who respectively found a frequency of 42.9% [110] and 41.6% [112] and higher than that of Fofana Y (23%) [113].

Seventy percent (70%) of our patients had dyslipidemia. This result was much higher than that of Mahamane Sani et al, who found 48.8% [107] but close to that of M.N. Munshi et al in the USA, who found a frequency of 77% [114].

These results could be explained by the diversity of people's lifestyles, urbanisation and, above all, sedentariness.

Arterial hypertension was associated with diabetes in 83.3% of our study. This result was similar to that found in the study by J. Doucet et al, in which it was 78% [115] and close to that of Mahamane Sani et al, who found 75.2% [107]; much higher than that found by Fofana Y and Dienta F, who found 61% [113] and 51.11% [106] respectively. This confirms what has been said in the literature on the fact that hypertension is a chronic disease frequently associated with diabetes either as a chronic complication or as a comorbidity. Calcium channel blockers were the most commonly used antihypertensive agents in our study, accounting for 36.6% of cases.

Duration of diabetes :

More than half the patients (53.3%) had developed diabetes for between 10 and 20 years. The mean duration of progression was 15 years. For the same age group, MA. Chami et al found a frequency of 31.4% [110]. Our results are in line with the literature, in which the majority of studies have shown that diabetes in the elderly is a form of diabetes that has been evolving for at least ten years.

Acute complications :

In our study, acute complications were mainly represented by hypoglycaemia (the most frequent according to the literature) and ceto-acidosis, each accounting for 13.3%. We found that hyperosmolarity, which according to the literature is the hallmark of T2DM, accounted for 6.7% of cases. Ikram S found a frequency close to ours for hypoglycemia in his study, 15.8% [115] compared with 7.53% for J.ABODO et al [108] and 81.5% for Mahamane Sani et al [107], who found a much higher frequency.

Chronic complications :

Peripheral neuropathy was the most common microangiopathic complication (53.3%), followed by diabetic retinopathy (46.6%). Fofana Y and Mahamane Sani et al found the same phenomenon but with widely different frequencies: respectively 50% and 79.5% for neuropathy; 21.40% and 32.1% for retinopathy.

diabétique [113, 107]. The divergence of these results in different studies could be explained by the divergence of socio-economic and demographic conditions (Mahamane Sani et al) for the performance of certain complementary examinations necessary for diagnosis, as well as the small size of our sample.

Infectious complications :

Infectious complications (pulmonary, digestive, cutaneous and urogenital) were present in 66.6% of our patients; this result was lower than that found by Mahamane Sani et al, who found an infectious frequency of 74.6% [107]. J.Doucet et al found an infectious frequency of 63%, dominated essentially by bronchopulmonary infections (35%) [116] as in our study (46.6%). This high frequency of infectious complications could be explained by the progressive decline in the immune defences of the elderly; the diversity in certain results is probably due to the much more unfavourable living conditions from one country to another.

5.7 According to the state of our patients at the overall geriatric assessment :

The majority of our patients were frail, 63.3% of cases; 20% were vigorous and 16.7% were dependent.

We found not only a statistical correlation between glycemic control and the age of our patients (p: 0.035), but also a statistical link between the same glycemic control and the state of our patients according to the global gerontological evaluation (p: 0.00).

In contrast to macoangiopathic complications, we found a statistically significant association between the occurrence of microangiopathic complications and the state of our patients according to their global gerontological assessment (P= 0.02).

5.8 Therapeutic aspects

More than half of our patients (63.33%) had insulin in their treatment regimen. This result was lower than those found by Ikram S and J ABODO et al who found a frequency of 77.6% and 90.2% respectively   [115, 108]. This could

In other words, this high frequency of insulin therapy can be explained by the decline in pancreatic function over the years, the contraindications to the use of OADs and the untimely onset of acute pathologies requiring transient insulin therapy.

Metformin was the most commonly used ADO in our study, with a frequency of 56.6%; antiaggregants were used with a frequency of 73.3% and statins were the most commonly used lipid-lowering treatment, accounting for 46.7% of cases.

Polymedication was statistically correlated with the state of our patients according to global geriatric evaluation (P= 0.008). The same observation was made by A. Trimeche et al at the Institut National de Nutrition Bab Saadoun in Tunisia, who found that polymedication accounted for 58% [117]. J. ABODO et al published an article in November 2019 on elderly diabetic subjects followed for 3 months in which he found a frequency of polymedication of 75.4% [108]. We found a frequency of 66.7% in our study.

PART VI

CONCLUSION

Our study involved 30 diabetic elderly subjects and we found a hospital frequency of 14.96% in our department. Type 2 diabetes, the most common type of diabetes, was found in 100% of our patients. Discovered during a work-up for polyuro-polydipsic syndrome in the majority of cases, it can be particularly disabling due to the occurrence of complications, especially in the elderly, in whom hypoglycaemia and infectious complications are frequent and can be formidable. It is most often associated with arterial hypertension, either as a macroangiopathic complication or as a comorbidity. Diabetes is a significant source of frailty, dependence and polymedication in the elderly, and its optimal management must be based on a progressive, multidisciplinary approach tailored to each patient (global geriatric assessment), involving in particular the diabetologist, geriatrician and general practitioner.

RECOMMENDATIONS :

To health authorities and political decision-makers:

Providing medical support for diabetics in state-run facilities and diabetes associations,

To disseminate information on sugar diabetes at the primary health care level, in order to educate the population by emphasising, among known diabetics, the means of avoiding acute metabolic complications and, among non-diabetics, the risk factors and primary symptoms of diabetes.

To the hospital's administrative authorities :

-Supplying pharmacies in ëtatic structures with mëdicament antidiabëtiques, especially gënëriques,

-Equipping the hospital laboratory to carry out certain emergency tests such as blood ionograms, blood gases, creatinine and CBC.

-To provide the internal medicine department with a permanent supply of dipsticks (urine and blood) and glucomëtre,

- Training healthcare workers in the technique of patient therapeutic education (ETP).

People with diabetes and their families:

-Accepting and understanding their illness,

-Observe hyggiëno-diëtëtic measures,

-Respect the dosage of medicines and the times at which they should be taken,

-Keep appointments йхёз for clinical and biological monitoring,

-Possëder a glucomëtre if possible.

To nursing staff:

-Dëpister all diabetic patients,

-Providing regular, appropriate care for diabetic patients,

-Providing therapeutic education for diabetic patients and their families.

REFERENCES

[1] Report of the Expert Committee on the Diagnosis and Classification of Diabetes Mellitus, Diabetes Care, July 1997. vol 20. n° 7, p. 1183-1197.

[2] Dusquesne F. Vuirarabiitis of the адёе person. Congres SFMU ; Urgences 2011, pp.277291

[3] Gёriatrie pour ie praticien, Beimin J, Chassagne P, Friocourt P, Gonthier R, Jeandei C, Nourhashёmi F, et ai, eds. Paris: Masson; 2009

[4] T. Mercer et al. Mitigating the Burden of Diabetes in Sub-Saharan Africa Through an Integrated Diagonai Heaith Systems Approach. Diabetes Metab. Syndr. Obes. Targets Ther. Oct 2019; 2261-2272.

[5] Fёdёration Internationaie du diabete. Atias du diabete. 9th ёdition Quebec. 2019.

[6] F.D. COULIBALY. Frequence et prise en charge des pieds diabёtiques dans ie service de medecine et d'endocrinologie de I'hopital du Mali. Thёse : Med : FMOS de Bamako. 2014 ; 101p.

[7] IIautc Autoritc dc Sante. Prescription for physical and sports activity for type 1 diabetes. Organisation des parcours. HAS; September 2018. URL: https://www.has-sante.fr/upioad/docs/appiication/pdf/2018-10/ref_aps_dt2_vf.pdf

[8] American Diabetes Association. 2. Diagnosis and Diagnosis of Diabetes: Standards of Medicai Care in Diabetes. Diabetes Care, Jan. 2018. voi. 41, n° Suppi. 1, p. S13-S27.

[9] Louis Monnier. Diabёtoiogie. 3^dition. Paris. March 2019.

[10] The World Health Organization (WHO). Definition and diagnosis of diabetes meiiitus and intermediate hypergiycemia. Report of a Worid Heaith Organization Consuitation. Diagnosis.   Eniigne   .   1965. p46.   Disponibie a
the
URL:https://apps.who.int/iris/bitstream/handie/10665/43588/9241594934_eng.pdf?sequence =1

[11] Bottazzo GF, Fiorin-Christensen A, Doniach D. Isiet-ceii antibodies in diabetes meiiitus with auto-immune poiyendocrine deficiencies. Lancet. 1974. 2. P. 1279-83.

[12] Christy M, Nerup J, Bottazzo GF, et al. Association between HLA-B8 and autoimmunity in juveniie diabetes. Lancet. 1976. 2. p.142-3.

[13] Marchand L, Thivolet C. Etiology and pathophysiology of type 1 diabetes. EMC. Endocrinologie. June 2016. 13(4) :1-12.

[14] Buffet et al. Endocrinologie, diabёtologie, nutrition. Issy-les-moulineaux Elsevicr Masson. 2010. 1. p 446.

[15] college des enseignants d'endocrinologie, diabete et maladies mёtaboliques. Endocrinologie, diabёtologie et maladies mёtaboliques Issy-les-Moulineaux cedex, France: Elsevier Masson. 2019. 4th ёd.

[16] De Fronzo RA, Bonadonna RC, Ferrannini E. Pathogenesis of NIDDM. A balanced overview. Diabetes Care. 1992. 15. p318-68.

[17] Diabetes Prevention Program Research Group. Reduction in the incidence of type 2 diabetes with lifestyle intervention or metformin. N Engl J Med. 2002. 346. p 393-403.

[18] Kahn BB, Flier JS. Obesity and insulin resistance. J Clin Invest .2000. 106. p 473-81.

[19] Kahn CR. Insulin action, diabetogenes, and the cause of type II diabetes. Diabetes .1994. 43. p 1066-84.

[20] Bergsten P. Pathophysiology of impaired pulsatile insulin release. Diabetes Metab Res

Rev. 2000. 16. p 179-91.

[21] O'Meara NM, Sturis J, van Cauter EV, Polonsky KS. Lack of control of ultradian insulin secretory oscillations in impaired glucose tolerance and innoninsulin- dependent diabetes mellitus. J Clin Invest .1993. 92. p 262-71.

[22] Polonsky KS, Given BD, Hirsch LJ, et al. Abnormal patterns of insulin secretion in noninsulin-dependent diabetes mellitus. N Engl J Med. 1988. 318. p 1231-9.

[23] Bratush-Marrain PR, Komjati M, Waldhausl WK. Efficacy of pulsatile-versus continuous insulin administration on hepatic glucose production and glucose utilization in type 1 diabetic humans. Diabetes care. 1986. 35. p 922-6.

[24] Cerasi E, Luft R. The plasma insulin response to glucose infusion in healthy subjects and in diabetes mellitus. Acta Endocrinol (Kbh). 1967. 55. p 278-304.

[25] Fujita Y, Herrow AL, Seltzer HS. Confirmation of impaired early insulin response to glycemic stimulus in non-obese mild diabetes. Diabetes care. 1975. 24. p 17-27.

[26] Pfeiffer MA, Halter JB, Porte D. Insulin secretion in diabetes mellitus. Am J Med. 1981. 70. p 579-88.

[27] Brunzell JD, Robertson RP, Lerner RL, et al. Relationship between fasting plasma glucose levels and insulin secretion during intravenous glucose tolerance tests. J Clin Endocrinol Metab. 1976. 42. p 222-9.

[28] obey FWJ, Beer SF, Carrington CA, et al. Sensitive and specific twosite immunoradiometric assays for human insulin, proinsulin, 65-66 split and 32-33 split proinsulins. Biochem J. 1989. 260. p 535-41.

[29] Davies M, Metcalfe J, Gray IP, et al. Insulin deficiency rather than hyperinsulinemia in newly diagnosed type 2 diabetes mellitus. Diabet Med. 1993. 10. p 305-12.

[30] Temple RC, Carrington GA, Luzio SD, et al. Insulin deficiency in noninsulin- dependent diabetes. Lancet. 1989. 1. p 293-5.

[31] Temple RC, Clark PMS, Nagi DK, et al. Radio immunoassay may overestimate insulin in non-insulin-dependent diabetics. Clin Endocrinol. 1990. 32. p 689-93.

[32] Levy J, Atkinson AB, Bell PM, et al. Beta-cell deterioration determines the onset and rate of progression of secondary dietary failure in type 2 diabetes mellitus: the 10-year follow-up of the Belfast Diet Study. Diabet Med. 1998. 15. p 290-6.

[33] UK Prospective Diabetes Study Group. U.K. Prospective Diabetes Study 16. Overview of 6 years therapy of type II diabetes: a progressive disease. Diabetes. 1995. 44. p 1249-58.

[34] Krauss S, Zhang CY, Scorrano L, et al. Superoxide-mediated activation of uncoupling protein 2 causes pancreatic в-cell dysfunction. J Clin Invest. 2003. 112. p 1831-42.

[35] Sakuraba H, Mizukami H, Yagihashi N, et al. Reduced beta-cell mass and expression of oxidative stress-related DNA damage in the islets of Japanese type II diabetic patients. Diabetologia. 2002. 45. p 85-96.

[36] Hod M, Kapur A, Sacks DA, Hadar E, Agarwal M, Di Renzo GC, et al. The International Federation of Gynecology and Obstetrics (FIGO) Initiative on gestational diabetes mellitus: A pragmatic guide for diagnosis, management, and care. Int J Gynaecol Obstet. Oct 2015. 131 Suppl 3. p 173-211.

[37] Immanuel J, Simmons D. Screening and treatment for earlyonset gestational diabetes aellitus: a systematic review and meta-analysis. Curr Diab Rep. Oct 2017. 2. 17(11):115.

[38] Borot S. Kleinclauss C. Penfornis A. Hyperosmolar coma. EMC (Elsevier Masson SAS, Paris), Endocrinologie-Nutrition. 10-366-H-30. 2007.

[39] American Diabetes Association. Diagnosis and classification of diabetes mellitus.

Diabetes Care. Jan 2014. 37 Suppl 1. p 81-90.

[40] Sigrist, S. Brandle, M. (2015). Hyperglycëmic emergencies in 1 adult. EMH Media. 15(33) : 723-728

[41] Kitabchi AE, Umpierrez GE, Miles JM, Fisher JN. Hyperglycemic crises in adult patients with diabetes. Diabetes Care 2009. 32. p 1335-43.

[43] Sigrist, S. Brandle, M. Hyperglycëmic emergencies in adults. EMH Media. 2015. 15(33). p 723-728.

[44] Intensive blood-glucose control with sulphonylureas or insulin compared with conventional treatment and risk of complications in patients with type 2 diabetes (UKPDS 33). UK Prospective Diabëtes Study (UKPDS) Group. Lancet 1998; vol 352: 837-53

[45] Halimi S. Hypoglycëmia in diabëtic patients. EMC - Endocrinology Nutrition 2016 ;13(1) :1-10

[46] Ardigo, S. Philippe, J. Hypoglycëmie et diabëte. Revue Mëdicale Suisse. 2008, 4 : 137682

[47] Berrebi, W. Diagnostics et therapeutiques du symptome a la prescription 8e ëd. Paris: Vuibert, 2018

[48] Orban J.-C., Ichai C. Complications metaboliques aiguc's du diabëte. Reanimation. 2008, 17 : 761-767.

[49] Monnier L. Diabetologie, Issy-les-Moulineaux cedex, France: Elsevier Masson, 2019, 3rd ed.

[50] Bondil P. La dysfonction erectile. Paris: John Libbey Euro text; 2003.p.1394.

[51] Knowler WC, Barrett-Connor E, Fowler SE, Hamman RF, Lachin JM, Walker EA, et al. Reduction in the incidence of type 2 diabetes with lifestyle intervention or metformin. N Engl J Med. 2002 Feb 7;346(6):393-403;

[52] Delyfer M.-N, Delcourt C. Epidemiology of diabetic rdtinopathy in international and French data. Medecine des maladies mdtaboliques. 2018, Vol.12-N°7: 553-8

[53] Gariani K, DE Seigneux A., Pechdre-Bertschi A., Philippe J., Martin P.-Y.   (). Diabetic nephropathy. Swiss Medical Journal. 2012, 8 : 473-9.

[54] Monnier L. Diabetologie, Issy-les-Moulineaux cedex, France: Elsevier Masson, 2019, 3rd ed.

[55] USRDS Annual Data Report: Epidemiology of Kidney Disease in the United States. Bethesda: National Institutes of Health, National Institute of Diabetes and Digestive and Kidncy Diseases, 2018 available at 1'URL: https://www.usrds.org/2018/view/Default.aspx, accessed 16 July 2019.

[56] Vodoin V., Karazivan P. La nephropathie diabetique : une sucree de complication.Le Medecin du Quebec. 2010, 45 : 49-55.

[57] Gariani K., DE Seigneux A., Pechdre-Bertschi A., Philippe J., Martin P.-Y. Diabetic nephropathy. Revue Medicale Suisse. 2012, 8 : 473-9.

[58] McFarlane P et al. (). Chronic kidney disease in diabetes. Can J Diabetes. 2018, 42: 201-9.

[59] Monnier L. Diabetologie, Issy-les-Moulineaux cedex, France: Elsevier Masson, 2019, 3rd ed.

[60] Grimaldi A. Guide pratique du diabdte. Issy-les-Moulineaux cedex, France: Elsevier Masson. 2009, 4th ed

[61] Ha Van G, Hartemann-Heurtier A, Gautier F, Haddad J, Bensimon Y, Ponseau W, Baillot J, Fourniols E, Koskas F, Grimaldi A. Endocrinologie-Nutrition Pied diabetique, EMC

(Elsevier Masson SAS), Paris, 2011, 10-20.

[62] Moxey PW, Gogalniceanu P, Hinchliffe RJ, Loftus IM, Jones KJ, Thompson MM, et al. Lower extremity amputations, a review of global variability in incidence. Diabet Med. 2011 Oct. 28(10) :1144 - 53 ;

[63] college of teachers of endocrinology, diabetes and metabolic diseases. Endocrinology, diabetology and metabolic diseases. Issy-les-Moulineaux cedex, France: Elsevier Masson, 2019, 4th ed

[64] Giuliano F, Droupy S. Dysfunction ёrecШe. EMC (Elsevier Masson SAS, Paris), progress in urology 2013, 23: 629-637.

[65] Phë V, Roupret M, Ferhi K, Traxer O, Haab F, Beley S. Etiology and management of ёrectile dysfunction in the diabeëtic patient. EMC (Elsevier Masson SAS, Paris), Progres en urologie 2009, 19 : 364-371

[66] PERLEMUTER L, SELAM J-L, COLLIN DE L'HORTET G. Abreg6s. Connaissances et pratique. Diabetes et maladies mëtaboliques. 4th edition. Paris: Editions Masson, 2003. 408p.

[67] Gallois P, Valtee J-P, Le Noc Y. L'observance des prescriptions mëdicales: quels sont les facteurs en cause? How l'aтёlюrer? Mëdecine. 2006 Nov ; 2(9) :402-6.

[68] BATTU Caroline. Nutritional management of an adult with type 2 diabetes. Actuals pharmaceutiques 2014, vol 53 : 57-60

[69] Priscille Tremblais et al. Guide des aliments-la nutrition (en ligne) 9novembre 2017- disponible a 1'URL : https://www.1anutrition.fr/bien-dans-sonassiette.

[70] BUYSSCHAERT Martin. Diabëtologie clinique, 4eme ëdition. Paris : Editions De Boeck Supërieur, 2011 : 199 p.136

[71] LE JEUNNE Claire, VITAL DURAND Denis, Doroz 2017, practical guide to mëdrugs. 36th ëdition. Paris: Maloine, 2016: 2048 p.

[72] Zinman B. The physiologic replacement of insulin. N Engl J Med 1989; 321: 363-70.

[73] Eisenbarth GS. Type 1 diabetes mellitus. A chronic auto-immune disease. N Engl J Med 1986; 314: 1360-8.

[74] Monnier L, Benichou M, Charra-Ebrard S, et al. An overview of the rationale for the pharmacological strategies in type 2 diabetes: from the evidence to new perspectives. Diabetes Metab 2005; 31: 101-9.

[75] Monnier L, Colette C. Failure of oral antidiabëtics at maximal toterate doses: which injectable treatments? Mëdecine des maladies Mëtaboliques 2016; 10: 121-30.

[76] Hedia S, Faouzi K. Congres internationnal de Mëdecine Pluridisciplinaire: Les nouveaux antidiabëtiques oraux en 2019;   21 Mars 2009 ; Gammarth. Gammarth : International family doctors Association; 2009.

[77] Berrebi, W. (2018). Diagnostics and therapeutics from symptom to prescription (8th ëd). Paris: Vuibert

[78] American Diabetes Association-European Association for the Study of Diabetes. Prise en gestion de 1'huayperglycemie chez les patients diabët iques de type2 [En ligne]. 2012 Jun [20/12/2018]; vol(6): [28 pages] Available at 1'URL: https://www.sfdiabete.org

[79] Manderau-Bruno L, Fosse-Edorth S. Prevalence of pharmacologically treated diabetes (all types) in France. Territorial and socio-economic disparities. BEH 2017; 27-8.

[80] Diabetes in the elderly adults. Diabetes Metab 2005; 31: 5S1-11.

[81] Verny C, Hervy MP. Le diabete du sujet age. Encycl Med Chir, Paris Elsevier. Endocrinologie Nutrition, 10: 1998, 6 p

[82] Kirkman MS, Jones Briscoe V, Clark N, et al. Diabetes in older adults; a consensus

report. JAGS 2012; 60: 2342-56.

[83] Bansal N, Dhaliwal R, Weinstock RS. Management of diabetes in the elderly. Med Clin N Am 2015; 99: 351-77.

[84] Bourdel-Marchasson I, Helmer C, Fagot-Campagna A, Dehail P, Joseph PA. Disability and quality of life in elderly people with diabetes. Diabetes Metab. 2007; 1: S66-74.

[85] Fried LP, Tangen CM, Walston J, Newman AB, Hirsch C, Gottdiener J, Seeman T, Tracy R, Kop WJ, Burke G, McBurnie MA; Cardiovascular Health Study Collaborative Research Group.Frailty in older adults: evidence for a phenotype.J Gerontol A BiolSci Med Sci. 2001; 56: 146-56.

[86] Haute Autorite de Sante. Comment reperer la fragilite en soins ambulatoires. (On line) available at 1'URL : http://www.has-sante.fr

[87] Folstein MF, Folstein SE, MC Hugh P. "Mini Mental State": a practical method for grading the cognitive state of patients for the clinician. J Psy Res, 1975, 12: 189-98.

[88] Katz S, Moskowitz AB, Jackson BA, et al. Studies of illness in the elderly. The index of ADL: a standardized measure of biological and psychological function. JAMA, 1963, 185: 914-9.

[89] Katz S, Downsns TD, Cash R, Groth RC. Progress in development of the index of ADL. Gerontologist, Spring 1970, part I: 20-30.

[90] Lawton MP, Brody EM. Assessment of older people: self-maintenance and instrumental activities of daily living. Gerontologist, 1969, 9: 179-86.

[91] Guigoz Y, Vellas B, Garry PJ. The Mini Nutritional Assessment (MNA): a practical assessment tool for grading the nutritional state of elderly patients. Facts Res Gerontol, 1994, (suppl 2), 15-32.

[92] Pinies JA, Cairo G, Gaztambide S, Vasquez JA. Course and prognosis of 132 patients with diabetic non ketototic hyperosmolar state. Diabetes & Metab, 1994, 20: 43-8.

[93] Malone ML, Gennis V, Goodwin JS. Characteristics of diabetic ketoacidosis in older versus younger adults. J Am Geriatr Soc, 1992, 40: 1100-4.

[94] Diabetes in the elderly adults. Diabetes Metab 2005; 31(Special issue. 2): 5S1-11.

[95] Shorr RI, Ray WA, Daugherty JR, et al. Individual sulfonylureas and serious hypoglycemia in older people. J Am Geriatr Soc, 1996; 44: 751-5.

[96] Broker P, Capriz-Ribiere F, Hieronimus S. Hypoglycëmies in aдё diabetic patients. La Revue du Gënëraliste et de la Gërontologie, 1997, 31: 9-13.

[97] Diabëtes in the elderly. Part 2. Diabetes Metab 2007; 33(Suppl. 1): S1-86.

[98] Diabetes in the elderly adults. Diabetes Metab 2005; 31(Special issue. 2): 5S1-11.

[99] American Diabetes Association. Older adults. Sec.10. in Standards of medical care in diabetes-2016. Diabetes Care 2016; (Suppl.1) S81-5.

[100] Vischer UM, Bauduceau B, Bourdel-Marchasson I, et al. A call to incorporate the prevention and treatment of geriatric disorders in the management of diabetes in the elderly. Diabetes Metab 2009; 35 : 168-77.

[101] Bansal N, Dhaliwal R, Weinstock RS. Management of diabetes in the elderly. Med Clin N Am 2015; 99: 351-77.

[102] Darmon P, Bauduceau B, Bordier L, et al. Position statement of the Sociëtë Francophone du Diabëte (SFD) on the mëdicamentous management of hyperglycëmia in the type 2 diabetic patient. Medecine des maladies mëtaboliques 2017; 11: 577-93.

[103] Inzucchi SE, Bergenstal RM, Buse JB, et al. Management of hyperglycaemia in type 2 diabetes: a patient-centered approach. Position statement of the American Diabetes

Association (ADA) and the European Association for the Study of Diabetes (EASD). Diabetologia 2012;55:1577-96.

[104]   Le diabete. Echantillon national representatif des personnes diabëtiques Entred 2007-2010 [On line]. Available at

THE URL: http://www.invs.sante.fr//publications/entred/entred-2007-2010/index.html.

[105]   Guide to the management of diabëtic aдë. Mëdecine des maladies mëtaboliques 2008; (2). Hors^rie 1.

[106]   Dienta F. Probtematique de la prise en charge du diabete sucre chez les sujets du 3 eme age dans les unites crees au compte de 1'approche Steps Wise a Bamako et Kati [Thëse].Mëdecine : Bamako, kati ; 2009. 91p.

[107]   Mahamane Sani MA, Ada A , Tchatath NNV, Daou M , Brah S, Andia A, Malam-Abdou B, Adehossi E.Particular^s du Diabete du Sujet Aдë de Plus de 60 Ans au Niger. Health Sci. Dis: Vol 19 (1) Suppl 1 Feb 2018.

[108]   J.ABODO, A LOKROU, P KOFFI-DAGO, F KOUASSI, A HUE, AJC AZOH, A DERBE, M SANOGO. Carac^ristiques diabëtologiques et gëriatriques du sujet diabëtique agë hospitalisë a Yopougon.Service d'endocrinologie-diabëtologie, CHU deYopougon, abidjan, Cote d'lvoire.Rev Int Sc Med 2013;15,2:64-68.

[109]   Sophie Bucher. Diabete de type II et sujets de plus de 65 ans non institutionalisës : prise en charge par les mëdecins gënëralistes en conditions de vie reelle - Suivi de cohorte. Endocrinology and metabolism. Universe Paris Saclay (COmUE), 2018.

[110]   Chami MA, Zemmour L, Midoun N, Belhadj M. Diabete sucre du sujet agë : la premiere enquete a^rienne Diabetesmellitus in the elderly: The first Algerian survey 2015 . Mëdecine des maladies Mëtaboliques March 2015;Vol. 9 - N°2: 210-215.

[111]   C. GEIST. Admission for alteration of the "general state" to the Service d'Accueil et de traitements des Urgences (SAU) of the Nouvel Hopital Civil de Strasbourg. 2013 September. *Available at: http://www.smf.org*

[112]   Khadija Diyane,Nawal El Ansari, Ghizlane El Mghari, Karim Anzid, and Mohamed Cherkaoui. Characteristics of the association type 2 diabetes and hypertension in the elderlyaged 65 and over service d'endocrinologie-diabëtologie du CHU de Marrakech, du mois de Novembre 2010 au mois de Juillet 2011. Pan African Medical Journal2013; 100:14.
Available at: http://www.panafrican-med-journal.com/content/article/14/100/full/

[113]   Fofana et al. Diabete du sujet agë en pratique hospitaliere a Bamako. 2014 March. *Available at: http://www.em-consulte.com*

[114]   Munshi MN, Segal AR, Slyne C, SamurAA, Brooks KM, Horton ES. Shortfalls of the use of HbA1C-derived eAG in older adults with diabetes 2015. Diabetes Res ClinPract 2015 Oct; 110(1):60-5.

[115]   Ikram S. Diabete du sujet age [These]. Medecine : Marrakech ; 2017. 184p

[116]   Doucet J, Bauduceau B, Le Floch P, Verny C. Gerodiab study: description of 985 type 2 diabetic patients aged over 70 years. DiabetesMetabA 2011 ; 37 :36-A108.

[117]   A. Trimeche, F. Ben Slama, H. Ben Amara, H. Ibrahim, L. Dahmouni, N. Daly, F. Ben Mami. La polymedication chez le diabetique age ; LA TUNISIE MEDICALE - 2013 ; Vol 91 (n°01) : 50 - 53.

Appendices

Survey form

Survey form I. Identity : N° fiche :.................... **Patient contact:**

First name(s): Surname: Age: Sex: 1-H _/_/_2-F _/_/_Residence: Ethnic group: Bambara/ _/_peulh _/_/soninké/ _/
Profession: housewife/ _/_farmer/ _/Sonrhai/ _/mianka/ _/boa/ _/Signing/ _/Clerk/ _/Malinké/ _/bozo/ _/maure/ _/Civil
servant: active/ _/retired/ _/Tamacheck/ _/senoufo/ _/Other.. Other...........................
Weight: Height: Waist circumference: BMI:............ 1- thin _/_/2- normal _/_/3- overweight _/_/4- moderately obese
/ _/5- severely obese _/_/6- morbidly obese _/_/**II. Date of admission:** / / **III. Reason for hospitalisation: IV.**
Date diabetes discovered: / / **V. Method of discovery:** 1-discovery by chance _/_/2- health check _/_/3-Acute
complication _/_/if so which.. 4-Chronic complication _/_/5-Other _/_/

VI. Type of diabetes: 1-type 1 _/_/2-type 2 _/_/3-secundary _/_/

VII. Follow-up: 1-regular _/_/2-Regular _/_/**VIII. Treated since discovery:** 1-Yes _/_/2-No _/_/**IX. Initial**
treatment: 1-diet _/_/2-ADO _/_/3-insulin _/_/4-other _/_/

X. Current treatment: 1-diet _/_/2-ADO _/_/3-insulin _/_/4-other _/_/**XI. Personal history:** 1-HTA _/_/2-Asthma _/_/
3-Sickle cell disease _/_/4-Cardiopathy _/_/5-Nephropathy _/_/6-Hepatopathy _/_/7-Overweight _/_/8-Obesitis _/
_/9-Dyslipidaemia _/_/10-Other / / 11 -Autoimmunity / _/**XII. Family history:** 1-Diabetes _/_/2-HTA _/_/3-
nephropathy _/_/4-sickle cell disease _/_/5-cardiopathy _/_/6-Asthma _/_/7-hepatopathy _/_/8-other _/_/9-Auto-
immunity/ _/**Risk factors for diabetes:** a. Non-modifiable: 1-age _/_/2-heredity _/_/
3 Sex _/_/b. Modifiable: 1-sedentary lifestyle _/_/2-obesity / / 3-dyslipidaemia _/_/

XIII. Cardiocirculatory risk factors: a. Non-modifiable: 1-age _/_/2-heredity _/_/3-sex _/_/b. modifiable: 1-HTA
_/_/2-obesity _/_/3-alcohol _/_/4- sedentary lifestyle _/_/6- dyslipidaemia / _/5-cigarette _/_/

XIV. Complications

AIGUES :

A. Hyperosmolarity 1-Yes _/_/2- No _/_/**B. Ketoacidosis** 1- Yes _/_/2-No _/_/**C. Hypoglycaemia** 1-Yes _/_/2- No _/_/
D. Lactic acidosis 1- Yes _/_/2-No _/_/

CHONICS :

A. Micro angiopathy: 1-Yes _/_/2-No _/_/a. **Retinopathy** 1-Yes _/_/2-No _/_/FO
:...
If present, stage of retinopathy: ....
Other:................................... b. **Nephropathy** 1-Yes _/_/2-No _/_/Microalbuminuria 1- Yes _/_/...............
No _/_/Proteinuria 1-Yes _/_/............. 2-No _/_/Creatinemia .... Clearance ....
ECBU..
If present, stage of nephropathy:... c. **Peripheral neuropathy** 1-Yes _/_/2-No _/_/
Reflexes:..
Monofilament :..
Paresthesia: 1-Yes / / .... 2-No _/_/
B. Macroangiopathy a. Stroke 1-Yes _/_/2-No _/_/
CT:...
b. MI 1-Yes _/_/2-No _/_/Cardiac enzymes:...
ECG:.. ....
Echocoeur :...
Coronary angiography: 1-Yes/ _/2-No/ _/**c. Arteriopathy** 1-Yes _/_/2-No _/_/IM Doppler:
.... **d. High blood pressure:** 1-Yes _/_/2-No _/_/.
C. Podiatric complications 1-Yes _/_/2-No _/_/If yes, grade (TEXAS):......... ... **Stage 1** 1-Yes _/_/2-No _/_/**Stage2**
1-Yes _/_/2-No _/_/**Stage3** 1-Yes _/_/2-No _/_/**Stage4** 1-Yes _/_/2-No _/_/**D. Infectious complications** 1- Yes _/_/2-
No _/_/If yes, which and if possible the site or triggering factor:..
XV. Paraclinical HbA1c: .... triglycerides: ....TSHus :.................. total cholesterol:
..................HDLc :..................LDLc :.........................
Natremia:.....................kalemia:.......................calcemia:.................
NFS : GR :........................GB :...........................PLQ :...................................
Tx Hb :.....................VGM :..................CCMH :.....................TCMH :..................... PNN :.......................PNE
:.......................PNB :....................LYMP :................MONO :...............
Search for secondary causes of diabetes 1-Yes _/_/2-No _/_/If yes, which
one:... **a. Pancreatopathy** 1- Yes _/_/2- No _/_/**b. Drug abuse** 1- Yes _/_/2-
No _/_/**c. Endocrinopathy** 1- Yes _/_/2- No _/_/1-Treated _/_/2- Untreated _/_/**XVI. Global geriatric assessment**
Cognitive problems: 1- Yes _/_/2- No _/_/**MMS score: ....**
Dementia 1-Yes _/_/2- No _/_/**Alzheimer's disease** 1-Yes _/_/2- No _/_/Autonomy: 1-Yes _/_/2- No _/**AIVQ/IADL**
score:.........................
Malnutrition 1- Yes _/_/2- No _/_/**MNA score:**....................
Depression-Anxiety 1- Yes _/_/2- No _/_/**Mini GDS score :**..............

Mobility and risk of falls:.. **Tests: unipodal station** 1- Yes $\underline{/\,/}$ 2-No $\underline{/\,/}$ **Timed Get up and Go** 1-Yes $\underline{/\,/}$ 2-No $\underline{/\,/}$ Polymedication 1- Yes $\underline{/\,/}$ 2- No $\underline{/\,/}$ **a. ADO** 1-Yes $\underline{/\,/}$ 2-No $\underline{/\,/}$ **b. INSULIN** 1-Yes $\underline{/\,/}$ 2-No $\underline{/\,/}$ **c. ANTIHYPERTENSE** 1-Yes $\underline{/\,/}$ 2-No $\underline{/\,/}$ **d. ANTALGIC** 1-Yes $\underline{/\,/}$ 2-No $\underline{/\,/}$ **e. NEUROLEPTIC** 1-Yes $\underline{/\,/}$ 2-No $\underline{/\,/}$ **f. PLAQUETARY ANTIAGGREGANT** 1-Yes $\underline{/\,/}$ 2-No $\underline{/\,/}$ **g. STATIN** 1-Yes $\underline{/\,/}$ 2-No $\underline{/\,/}$ **h. ANTIARTHMIC** 1-Yes $\underline{/\,/}$ 2-No $\underline{/\,/}$ **i. ANTIBIOTIC** 1-Yes $\underline{/\,/}$ 2-No $\underline{/\,/}$ **Drugs** ....
....

Global geriatric assessment form

TEST DE FOLSTEIN ou Mini Mental Score (MMS)

1. ORIENTATION TEMPS ET ESPACE (1 point par réponse exacte)

En quelle année sommes nous ?
Quelle saison ?
Quel mois ?
Quelle est la date ?
Quel est le jour de la semaine ?

Dans quelle ville sommes nous ?
Dans quel département ?
Dans quelle région ?
Quel est le nom de la rue ?
Quel est le nom de la pièce où nous sommes ?

SCORE (maximum 10)

2 . APPRENTISSAGE

Donner 3 noms d'objets usuels (chaussure, fleur, porte)
Compter 1 point par mot correctement répété au 1er essai

SCORE (maximum 3)

3 . ATTENTION ET CALCUL

Demander de compter, à partir de 100, en retirant 7 à chaque fois
Arrêter après 5 soustractions. Noter le nombre de réponse correcte

SCORE (maximum 5)

Si le patient refuse (score 0) , on lui demande d'épeler le mot MONDE
à l'envers. 1 point par lettre en bonne place

SCORE MONDE (maximum 5)

4 . RAPPEL - MEMOIRE

Demander les 3 noms d'objets présentés auparavant
(1 Point par réponse correcte)

SCORE (maximum 3)

5 . LANGAGE

Monter et demander le nom : stylo et montre (1point par item)
Faire répéter : "il n'y a pas de mais ni de si ni de et " : 1point ou 0
Faire exécuter un ordre triple : prenez cette feuille de papier, pliez la et
jetez la par terre (1 point par item correct)
Faire lire et exécuter un ordre écrit : "fermez les yeux " : 1 point ou 0
Ecriture spontanée : une phrase. Ne pas donner d'exemple
(1 point pour une phrase simple. Orthographe et grammaire indifférentes)

Faire copier le dessin suivant :
1 point si les 2 polygones sont
corrects et entrecoupés au niveau
de leur angle droit
NB : Ce test est trés sensible aux atteintes organiques uébutantes

SCORE (maximum 9)

SCORE TOTAL (Maximum 30) :
RESULTATS
—— Un score total de 30 permet de rassurer le patient.
—— Entre 20 et 30, le diagnostic ne peut être posé, compléter les explorations.
— Au dessous de 20, il existe un réel trouble

Mobilité et risque de chute

Up & Go test

Inviter la personne à :	Fait : 1	Ne fait pas : 0	Non réalisable
• Se lever d'un fauteuil avec accoudoirs :	☐	☐	☐
• Traverser la pièce - distance de 3 mètres :	☐	☐	☐
• Faire demi-tour :	☐	☐	☐
• Revenir s'asseoir :	☐	☐	☐

• Temps nécessaire : _____ secondes.
• Score : _____ / 4

Interprétation : risque de chute si score ≤ 1 et temps de réalisation > 20 secondes.
On note également les lenteurs d' exécution, les hésitations, une marche trébuchante.

Test Unipodal

Demander à la personne de rester en appui sur 1 pied sans aide pendant au moins 5 secondes.

	Oui	Non	Non réalisable
• Pied droit :	☐	☐	☐

• Pied gauche :

Echelle des activités instrumentales de la vie quotidienne - Test de Lawton   ☐

Activités		Cotation femmes	Cotation hommes
1. Téléphone	Utilise le téléphone de sa propre initiative, compose le numéro	1	1
	Compose quelques numéros connus	1	1
	Décroche mais ne compose pas seul	1	1
	N'utilise pas le téléphone	0	0
2. Faire les courses	Achète seul la majorité des produits nécessaires	1	1
	Fait peu de courses	0	0
	Nécessite un accompagnement lors des courses	0	0
	Incapable de faire ses courses	0	0
3. Faire la cuisine	Prévoit et cuisine les repas seul		1
	Cuit les repas après préparation par une tierce personne		0
	Fait la cuisine mais ne tient pas compte des régimes imposés		0
	Nécessite des repas préparés et servis		0
4. Ménage	S'occupe du ménage de façon autonome		1
	Fait seul des tâches ménagères légères		1
	Fait les travaux légers mais de façon insuffisante		1
	Nécessite de l'aide pour les travaux ménagers		1
	Nécessite de l'aide pour les travaux ménagers quotidiens		0
5. Linge	Lave tout son linge seul		1
	Lave le petit linge		1
	Tout le linge doit être lavé à l'extérieur		0
6. Transport	Utilise les moyens de transport de manière autonome	1	1
	Commande et utilise seul un taxi	1	1
	Utilise les transports publics avec une personne accompagnante	0	0
	Parcours limités en voiture, en étant accompagné	0	0
	Ne voyage pas	0	0
7. Médicaments	Prend ses médicaments correctement et de façon responsable	1	1
	Prend correctement les médicaments préparés	0	0
	Ne peut pas prendre les médicaments correctement	0	0
8. Argent	Règle ses affaires financières de façon autonome	1	1
	Règle ses dépenses quotidiennes, aide pour les virements et dépôts	1	1
	N'est plus capable de se servir de l'argent	0	0

Pour chaque item, la cotation ne peut être que 0 et 1. Le score est côté de 0 à 5 pour les hommes et de 0 à 8 pour les femmes. 0 désignant une dysautonomie totale et 8 une personne totalement autonome

Dépistage de l'état nutritionnel MNA (Mini Nutritional Assessment)		
Le patient a-t-il mangé moins des 3 derniers mois par manque d'appétit, problèmes digestifs, difficultés de mastication ou de déglutition ? 0 anorexie sévère 1 anorexie modérée 2 = pas d'anorexie		..... Pts
Perte récente de poids (<3 mois) : 0 perte de poids > 3 kg 1 ne sait pas 2 = perte de poids entre 1 et 3 kg 3 = pas de perte de poids		..... Pts
Motricité : 0 du lit au fauteuil 1 autonome à l'intérieur 2 sort du domicile		..... Pts
Maladie aiguë ou stress psychologique lors des 3 derniers mois ? 0 = oui 2 = non		..... Pts
Problèmes neuropsychologiques : 0 démence ou dépression sévère 1 démence ou dépression modérée 2 = pas de problème psychologique		..... Pts
Indice de masse corporelle IMC (IMC = poids/(taille^2) en kg/m^2) : 0 IMC < 19 1 IMC entre 19 et 21 2 = IMC entre 21 et 23 3 = IMC >23		..... Pts
Score de dépistage (max 14 pts) 12 pts au plus : normal 11 pts ou moins : malnutrition possible (faire appel à la diététicienne)		1 .. Pts

Dépistage de la dépression chez la personne âgée (mini-GDS)

Pour des scores de mini GDS ≥ 1, la probabilité de dépression est forte (sensibilité : 88%, spécificité : 63%) et il convient d'utiliser l'échelle de dépression gériatrique de 15 points

Vous sentez vous souvent découragé et triste?	oui =1 / non=0
Avez-vous le sentiment que votre vie est vide?	oui =1 / non=0
Êtes vous heureux (se) la plupart du temps?	oui =0 / non=1
Avez-vous l'impression que votre situation est désespérée ?	oui =1 / non=0

FACT SHEET

Last name: BAGAYOGO   **First name :** Lassine **City:** Bamako

Country of origin : Mali   **Telephone :** (00223) 75494348

Email address : lbagayogo95@gmail.com **Year of defence : 2022-2023**

Title of thesis: Epidemiological, clinical and therapeutic aspects of diabetes in the elderly in the internal medicine department of the CHME "LE LUXEMBOURG".

Areas of interest: Internal medicine, diabetology and geriatrics.

Depository: Library of the Faculty of Medicine and Odontostomatology.

SUMMARY :

Introduction: Diabetes in the elderly is a particularly sensitive subject that has received little attention in the literature. It is a fairly complex entity, given the physiological ageing process, with the concepts of polypathology and polymecation linked, among other things, to age, and the polymorphism of diabetes itself. Its management requires an individualised, patient-centred approach, with the prior definition of objectives based on an overall geriatric assessment.

Method: This was an observational, descriptive, cross-sectional study with prospective data collection carried out between 01 July 2020 and 31 December 2020 (six (6) months) on 30 patients in the internal medicine department of the CHME "LE LUXEMBOURG".

Objectives: To study the epidemiological, clinical and therapeutic aspects of diabetes in the elderly in the internal medicine department of the Centre Hospitalier Mere-Enfant (CHME) le Luxembourg in Bamako.

Results: The mean age was 75.23, with extremes ranging from 65 to 90 years, and the sex ratio was 1. We found a hospital frequency of 14.97%, with alteration of general condition the most common reason for hospitalisation (26.7%). All our patients were type 2 diabetics, i.e. 100%; 86.7% of them were discovered during an assessment of the polyuro-polydipsic syndrome, and all had at least 1 non-modifiable risk factor for diabetes and cardiovascular disease.Acute complications were mainly hypoglycaemia and cetoacidosis (13.3 each); peripheral neuropathy was the most common microangiopathic complication (53.3%), followed by diabetic retinopathy (46.6%); infectious complications were mainly pulmonary infection (63.6%). Arterial hypertension was associated with diabetes in 83.3% of cases, either as a macroangiopathic complication or as a comorbidity, and was treated with a CI in 36.6% of cases.63.3% of our patients were frail, 20% were vigorous and 16.7% dependent; 63.33% had insulin in their treatment regimen, and metformin was the most commonly prescribed OAD, accounting for 56.6% of cases. Sixty-six point seven of the patients (66.7%) were polymedic.

KEYWORDS: Diabetes, elderly, internal medicine, CHME

DATA SHEET

Name: BAGAYOGO   **First name:** Lassine   **City:** Bamako

Country of origin : Mali **Telephone :** (00223) 75494348

Email address : lbagayogo95@gmail.com **Defense year:** 2022-2023

Title of the thesis: Epidemio-clinical and therapeutic aspects of diabetes in the elderly in the internal medicine Department of the CHME "LE LUXEMBOURG

Area of interest: Internal medicine, diabetology and geriatrics.

Place of deposit: Library of the Faculty of Medicine and Odonto-Stomatology.

SUMMARY:

Introduction: Diabetes in the elderly is a particularly sensitive subject and little addressed in studies. It is a fairly complex entity given physiological aging with the notions of polypathology and polymecation linked, among other things, to age and the polymorphism of diabetes itself. Its management requires an individualized approach, centered on the patient with the prior definition of objectives based on the global geriatric assessment.

Method: This was an observational, descriptive cross-sectional study with a prospective collection of data carried out between July 01, 2020 and December 31, 2020 (six (6) months) involving 30 patients in the internal medicine department. of the CHME "LUXEMBOURG".

Objectives: To study the epidemiological, clinical and therapeutic aspects of diabetes in the elderly in the internal medicine department of the Mother-Child Hospital Center (CHME) Luxembourg in Bamako

Results: The average age was 75.23 with extremes ranging from 65 to 90 years and the sex ratio was 1. We found a hospital frequency of 14.97% with the most frequently found reason for hospitalization, the deterioration of the general state, that is to say 26.7%. All of our patients were type 2 diabetics, i.e. 100%; discovered during a review of the polyuro-polydipsic syndrome in 86.7%, all presenting at least 1 non-modifiable risk factor for diabetes and cardiovascular disease. Acute complications were mainly marked by hypoglycemia and ketoacidosis, i.e. 13.3 each. Peripheral neuropathy was the most found microangiopathic complication, i.e. 53.3%, followed by diabetic retinopathy (46.6%). Infectious complications were mainly pulmonary infection, i.e. 63.6% . Arterial hypertension was associated with diabetes in 83.3% either as a macroangiopathic complication or as a comorbidity and was treated with an IC in 36.6 of cases. The majority of our patients were fragile, 63.3% of cases, 20 % were vigorous and 16.7% dependent; 63.33% had insulin in their treatment regimen, metformin was the most prescribed ADO, i.e. 56.6% of cases. Sixty-six point seven of the patients (66.7%) were polymedicated.

KEY WORDS: Diabetes, elderly, Internal medicine, CHME

HIPPOCRATIC OATH

In the presence of the masters of this faculty, of my dear fellow students, before the effigy of Hippocrates, I promise and swear in the name of the supreme being, to be faithful to the laws of honour and probity in the practice of medicine.

I will give free care to the needy and will never demand a salary above my work. I will not take part in any clandestine sharing of fees.

Admitted to the interior of houses, my eyes will not see what goes on there, my tongue will keep silent about the secrets entrusted to me and my status will not serve to corrupt morals or encourage crime.

I will not allow considerations of religion, nation, race, party or social class to come between my duty and my patient. I will respect human life from the moment of conception.

Even under threat, I will not use my medical knowledge against the laws of humanity.

Respectful and grateful to my teachers, I will give back to their children the education I received from their father.

May men esteem me if I am faithful to my promises! May I be shamed and despised by my colleagues if I fail to do so.

I swear!

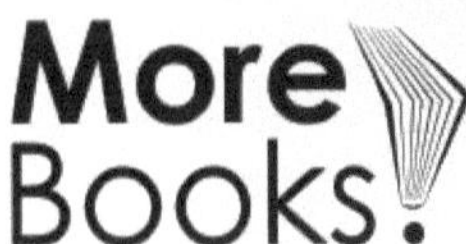

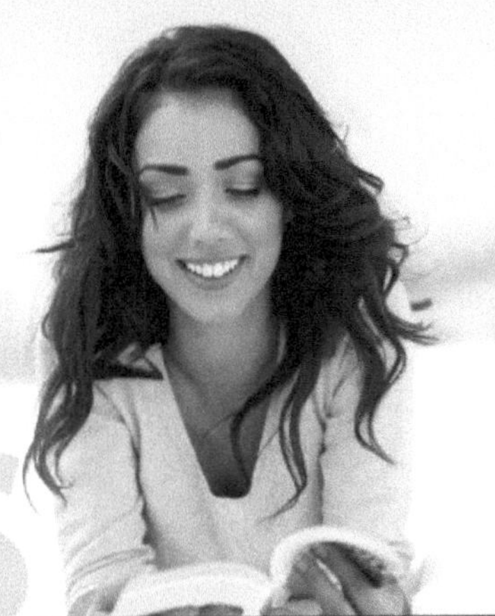

I want morebooks!

Buy your books fast and straightforward online - at one of world's fastest growing online book stores! Environmentally sound due to Print-on-Demand technologies.

Buy your books online at
www.morebooks.shop

Kaufen Sie Ihre Bücher schnell und unkompliziert online – auf einer der am schnellsten wachsenden Buchhandelsplattformen weltweit! Dank Print-On-Demand umwelt- und ressourcenschonend produziert.

Bücher schneller online kaufen
www.morebooks.shop

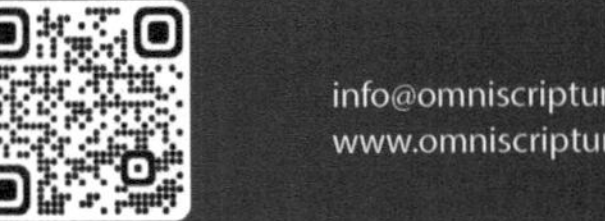

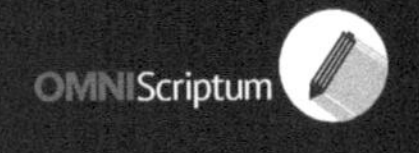

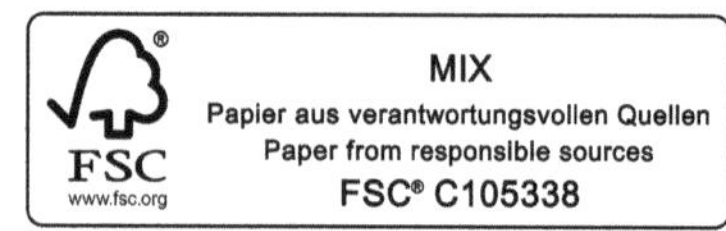

Printed by Books on Demand GmbH, Norderstedt / Germany